W9-COR-643

# *Living with Hepatitis C*

# Living with Hepatitis C

## Everything You Need to Know

Jenny Heathcote, MD
Colina Yim, RN
Quynh Thai, RN
Averell Sherker, MD

FIREFLY BOOKS

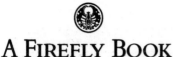

# A FIREFLY BOOK

Published by Firefly Books (U.S.) Inc. 2001

Copyright © 2001 by Jenny Heathcote

All rights reserved. No part of this publication may be reproduced, stored in a retrieval system or transmitted in any form or by any means, electronic, mechanical, photocopying, recording or otherwise, without the prior written permission of the publisher.

First Printing

U.S. CATALOGING-IN-PUBLICATION DATA
(Library of Congress Standards)

Heathcote, Jenny.
   Living with hepatitis C : everything you need to know /
Jenny Heathcote; Colina Yim; Quynh Thai; Averell Sherker. – 1st ed.
138 p. : cm. (Your personal health)
Includes index.
Summary: Understanding hepatitis C and its treatment.
ISBN: 1-55209-612-2 (pbk.)
1. Hepatitis C virus – Popular works. 2. Hepatitis C virus – Treatment
– Popular works. I Yim, Colina. II. Thai, Quynh. III. Sherker, Averell.
IV. Title. II. Series.
616.3623 21    CIP    QR201.H46H43 2001

Published in the United States in 2001 by
Firefly Books (U.S.) Inc.
P.O. Box 1338, Ellicott Station
Buffalo, New York, USA
14205

Published in Canada in 2001 by Key Porter Books Limited.

Design: Peter Maher
Electronic formatting: Heidy Lawrance Associates

Printed and bound in Canada

# Contents

# Introduction

If you have just discovered that you have hepatitis C, take a deep breath and relax for a moment. You are not alone—nearly 1 in every 100 people in North America has been infected with hepatitis C. You are one of the few (30 percent) who have been identified. In fact, most people who are infected with hepatitis C don't even know that they are. You may have been diagnosed because you have symptoms, or perhaps you feel quite well and your infection was identified during a routine checkup. However you found out, it is always a shock to know that you have an infection that may cause you to have liver disease that can be severe enough eventually to require a liver transplant. Fortunately, liver replacement is only necessary in a minority of cases. The number seems large because the total number of persons with chronic infection is so large: approximately 250,000 to 300,000 in Canada, close to 3 million in the U.S.A. and many millions worldwide.

One of the helpful ways to come to terms with your infection is to understand more about hepatitis C. There are many ways to gain information in these high-tech times, but it is important to ensure that the information is reliable, not just a personal opinion or observation. This book has been written by a team of physicians and nurses who have spent several years working with people infected with hepatitis C. Collectively we have listened to thousands of infected individuals from all walks of life. We have all actively participated in clinical research studies where new therapies are evaluated. We all have an ongoing interest in understanding why and how hepatitis C does what it does.

We hope that this book will help you understand the current state of knowledge regarding hepatitis C: how it can affect your body, how you can prevent spreading the infection, and what treatments you may want to consider.

# O N E

## *The Liver and Hepatitis*

The liver is the largest organ in our bodies. In an adult, it weighs between 2.5 and 3.5 pounds (1200 to 1500 gm). It lies in the upper right-hand side of the abdomen, mostly hidden under the ribcage, separated from the right lung by the diaphragm. The liver is shaped rather like a pyramid lying on its side.

The liver is made up of two main lobes, the left and the right. These are further subdivided into a total of eight segments, based on the liver's blood supply. There are billions of individual cells within the liver, the most common being the *hepatocytes*, which are arranged in an orderly fashion in units known as *lobules*.

## What Does the Liver Do?

Blood going through the liver flows between the liver cells, delivering oxygen, other necessary foodstuffs and material to be eliminated from the body. At the same time, proteins and other substances manufactured by the liver cells are taken up into the blood. There are areas called *portal tracts* between all the liver lobules. The portal tracts contain three different structures: the portal vein and the *hepatic artery*, which carry blood into the liver lobule, and the *bile duct*, which carries bile out of the lobule.

**Liver in abdomen**

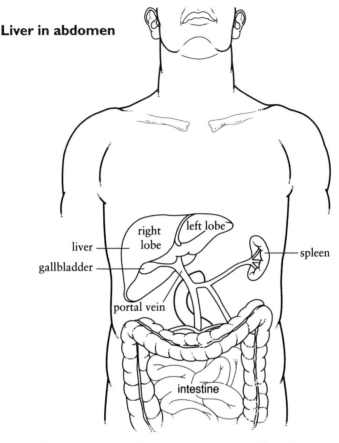

The liver is unique because it receives blood—containing vital oxygen—from two sources rather than one. Most of its blood flow is supplied through the low-pressure portal vein, which also collects blood rich in nutrients from the intestine and delivers the nutrients to the liver for processing. About a quarter of its blood flow is derived from the hepatic artery, and this artery's main function is to supply most of the oxygen that the liver requires for all the work it has to do. The liver *sinusoids*—spaces for blood to flow between the cords of liver cells—flow into veins that drain blood from the liver back to the heart.

## Lobules

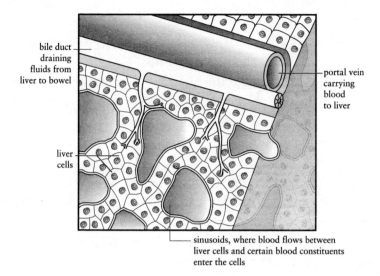

bile duct draining fluids from liver to bowel

portal vein carrying blood to liver

liver cells

sinusoids, where blood flows between liver cells and certain blood constituents enter the cells

The liver plays a critical role in the formation of proteins, carbohydrate and fat—the three essential components of the body. It makes most of the proteins that circulate in the bloodstream, which are required for normal blood clotting as well as for many other important functions. It keeps the blood sugar at a steady level by storing glucose (from food) as glycogen and releasing it when we need it for energy. Without this balancing, our blood sugar would fall to dangerously low levels overnight or even between meals. Cholesterol is manufactured in the liver. Although too much of a certain type of cholesterol can be a bad thing, cholesterol is an essential component of all the cells in the body. As well, the liver is the main organ in the body that breaks down toxins, drugs and alcohol, which are then eliminated in the bile.

Bile is made in the hepatocytes and drains into the biliary system, which looks like a tree with millions of branches. The tips of the smallest branches are at the liver cells, and the "trunk" where they eventually come together is the bile duct. There is a side arm of the bile duct—the gallbladder—where bile is stored and concentrated before it is released. Additionally, bile salts ("human detergents") are produced in the liver and drain through the biliary system into the intestine. Without the bile salts in bile we would be unable to digest and absorb fats and some essential vitamins.

## What Is Hepatitis?

Hepatitis simply means inflammation of the liver. It can be caused by any one of a large number of factors, including a virus infection, alcohol and drugs, as well as some metabolic conditions, such as those that cause too much fat to be deposited in the liver.

Most often, hepatitis is without symptoms and can only be detected through blood tests. However, hepatitis can cause symptoms that include fatigue, yellow discoloration of the skin and eyes (*jaundice*), nausea, loss of appetite and pain in the upper abdomen.

Physicians often use the terms *acute hepatitis* or *chronic hepatitis*. By definition, if the hepatitis lasts for more than six months it is chronic (persistent). Virus infections of the liver may be short-lived or chronic, depending on the type of infecting virus and also, in part, on the individual's response to the infection. It is important to realize that the term "chronic" relates only to the duration of the hepatitis, and does not imply anything about the severity of the process.

## What Is a Virus?

Viruses are infectious agents that are best thought of as incomplete organisms. They lack the machinery required to reproduce themselves and must enter the cells of other organisms—animals or plants—to multiply. They "pirate" the enzymes of the cells they infect to produce their genetic material and proteins, which can then be released from these cells into the circulation of the animal or plant.

Some viruses have relatively little effect on their hosts, while others can kill the cells they infect. A virus can also act as a target or "lightning rod" for the host's immune cells, called *lymphocytes*, and can even cause these lymphocytes to damage or destroy the host cells infected by the virus.

Many viruses persist in the body for a long time—even for the rest of the host's life. Some can enter a dormant or sleeping phase, and have the potential to become reactivated at certain times. Viruses tend to have very specific requirements for them to multiply, so they cannot grow in all cells or in certain animals. Some viruses can change the function of the cells that they infect, and promote the development of cancer.

## What Are the Viruses That Cause Hepatitis?

An infectious disease characterized by jaundice has been recognized for centuries—in fact, there is reference to the occurrence of jaundice in ancient Chinese, Babylonian, Greek and Roman literature. Epidemics were frequent, particularly among the military, and the condition came to be known as campaign jaundice. It was only in the late nineteenth century that it was recognized that jaundice might be caused by an infectious agent. In the 1930s it was observed that jaundice frequently occurred after exposure to others with jaundice, supporting the idea that an infectious agent could be the cause. During World War II, human volunteers were used to prove that hepatitis could be caused by viruses. During this time, it was recognized that there were two distinct patterns of transmission of viral hepatitis: by feces or by blood. In 1947, an English physician, Dr. MacCallum, coined the terms *hepatitis A* and *hepatitis B*.

## Hepatitis A

Hepatitis A, or infectious hepatitis, has a short incubation period. The time between exposure to the virus and onset of illness is only two to four weeks. It is spread through food or drinking water contaminated with the feces (stools) of infected persons, and tends to occur in epidemics.

## Hepatitis B

Hepatitis B has a longer incubation period (up to six months) and appears to be spread by exposure to blood and by sexual contact.

In 1963, the American biochemist Baruch Blumberg made a discovery for which he would eventually be awarded the Nobel Prize. He found something in the blood of an Australian Aborigine that reacted specifically with an antibody in the blood of an American patient who had received many transfusions because he had hemophilia (a blood clotting disorder). This "something" was a protein that Blumberg called the *Australia antigen*, which was found to be rare in North American and Western European populations, but was common among Asian and African populations, as well as among certain institutionalized persons, and people who had had frequent exposure to blood products. By 1967 it was recognized that Australia antigen was the protein that coated the surface of the hepatitis B virus, and this protein was renamed hepatitis B surface antigen (HBsAg). This antigen can be detected using blood tests, and since 1971 all blood donors in North America and most of the developed world have been tested for HBsAg. This strategy has proven very effective in reducing the spread of hepatitis B virus.

A major breakthrough has been the development of effective vaccines to prevent infection with hepatitis A virus and hepatitis B virus. The appropriate use of these vaccines has the potential to prevent virtually all new infections.

## Other hepatitis viruses

*Hepatitis D virus*, or the *delta agent*, is an "incomplete virus"—that is, it can only cause disease in people who are also infected with another virus, in this case hepatitis B virus. It may be responsible for both more severe acute hepatitis and chronic hepatitis. Infection with this virus is largely limited to specific geographic areas, including southern regions of Italy and parts of South America. In North America, hepatitis D virus is most commonly seen among intravenous drug users who have hepatitis B. Although there is no specific vaccine for this virus, effective use of hepatitis B virus vaccine will eliminate the risk for hepatitis D virus infection, as the latter cannot survive without hepatitis B.

*Hepatitis E virus* was discovered in the late 1980s. It is likely the most common cause of viral hepatitis worldwide but is virtually nonexistent in countries of the developed world. Like hepatitis A virus, it is spread through fecal contamination, and it has been responsible for massive epidemics in Asia and Central America. Epidemics typically occur in rainy seasons when the usual sanitation measures break down. Hepatitis E virus causes acute hepatitis that is of limited duration. Death is rare except in pregnant women, although the reasons for this particular increased death rate are not clear. To date, there is no vaccine to prevent hepatitis E virus infection.

There have been recent reports of novel hepatitis viruses, particularly *hepatitis G virus* and a virus named *TTV*. The importance of these remains to be fully discovered, but to date they do not appear to be important causes of serious acute or chronic liver disease.

Additionally, a large number of viruses that typically infect other organs of the body can have transient effects on the liver. These tend to cause mild liver disease in most cases. Among them are the Epstein-Barr virus (responsible for infectious mononucleosis), cytomegalovirus, herpes simplex virus, varicella (responsible for chickenpox and shingles) and human immunodeficiency virus (HIV, the AIDS virus).

## Hepatitis C

Soon after the discovery of these two hepatitis viruses, it became obvious that many cases of hepatitis—particularly those that occurred following a blood transfusion—were due to neither hepatitis A nor hepatitis B. By the mid-1970s, the term "non-A, non-B hepatitis" had been coined for the virus presumed responsible for these infections. It took over a decade before the hepatitis C virus was identified and found to be the cause of the vast majority of "non-A, non-B hepatitis" infections. These days, donated blood can be tested for the hepatitis C antibody. More recently it has become possible to test for the virus itself, but such testing is still far from universal.

The discovery of the hepatitis C virus has made it possible to specifically identify most people who have a viral infection affecting their liver. It would be even better if we could prevent this infection. However, we still have no vaccine to prevent hepatitis C. Moreover, people who have recovered from hepatitis C do not gain immunity, as happens in some diseases; if they are exposed to the virus again, they may become infected again. So until we do have a vaccine, people will continue to become infected, and the disease will not disappear. Most hepatitis C infections persist, often for a lifetime, unless antiviral therapy is successful. Hepatitis C is one of the most common liver diseases in the United States and Canada, and in most countries in the Western world.

## Identifying the Hepatitis C Virus

With the recognition of the impact of non-A, non-B hepatitis in the 1970s, there was an intensive worldwide effort to identify the virus responsible. The breakthrough came in 1988, when scientists at Chiron Corporation in California, using sensitive state-of-the-art molecular biology techniques, cloned (reproduced) a portion of the virus from the blood of a chimpanzee that had been experimentally infected with the virus from the blood of a human with non-A, non-B hepatitis. This virus was named hepatitis C virus. Then a test was developed to detect antibodies in the blood to this agent. It was shown that the vast majority of people diagnosed as having non-A, non-B hepatitis—especially those who had had exposure to blood or blood products—had antibodies to

## Inside the hepatitis C virus

The hepatitis C virus has been completely cloned and characterized in several laboratories around the world. It is spherical, with a diameter of approximately 50 nanometers (one two-hundredth of the diameter of a human hair). The virus has been found to contain ribonucleic acid (RNA) as its genetic material, or *genome*. The RNA genome of hepatitis C is approximately 9,500 nucleotide bases in length. About 9,000 of these nucleotides "code" for the proteins of the virus, while there are parts at either end of the genome that are involved in regulating the reproduction of the virus. The genome codes the three proteins that surround the virus, and the six (or more) proteins contained within the virus that allow it to multiply.

hepatitis C virus in their blood. By 1990, all blood donors were being tested for hepatitis C antibodies. Those who tested positive for hepatitis C antibody were excluded from the donor pool, and this has almost eliminated the risk of hepatitis C transmission by blood transfusion.

### How Does Hepatitis C Multiply and Remain in the Body?

As hepatitis C is a single-stranded RNA virus, it can only multiply by making a "complementary" or opposite RNA copy of itself, which in turn makes another complementary copy of itself, duplicating the original genome. An enzyme is required for hepatitis C virus to be able to make copies of itself, and this enzyme is called RNA-dependent RNA polymerase. This viral RNA polymerase is somewhat less reliable than the DNA polymerase found in human cells and is thus more prone to make mistakes. Paradoxically, these mistakes help the virus to avoid the immune system and survive in the body.

Our immune systems eliminate infections by recognizing them as being foreign to the body and destroying them. As the replication machinery of the hepatitis C virus often makes mistakes, the virus undergoes subtle changes that help to confound the immune system, and allow the changed virus to persist in the liver. This results in a mixed population of virus in the liver and blood of people infected with hepatitis C. The disparate sequences are known as *quasispecies*.

### Hepatitis C Genotypes and Subtypes

When viruses differ in approximately one-third of their genomic sequence, they are said to represent different *genotypes*. Just as species of animals have evolved over the millennia, the subtle changes that occur in the hepatitis C virus have resulted in different genotypes. It is recognized that there are at least six different hepatitis C virus genotypes—numbered 1 through 6. Less dramatic differences are found among viral *subtypes*.

Various hepatitis C viral genotypes predominate in different regions of the world. Genotype 1 (particularly subtype 1b) accounts for the majority of cases in North America, with genotypes 2 and 3 making up almost all the other cases. There are conflicting data about the severity of disease caused by different genotypes. The major clinical reason for identifying the genotype is to help us determine the appropriate duration of antiviral treatment, when it is indicated. This will be discussed in Chapter 5.

## What Does Hepatitis C Virus Do to the Liver?

Hepatitis C virus enters the body through the bloodstream and finds its way to the liver, where it enters the liver cells. Its viral genome gains access to the cellular machinery of the hepatocyte, so it is able to multiply its genome and make the proteins the virus requires. Viral particles then leave the liver cells and re-enter the bloodstream, or spread to other liver cells. Hepatitis C virus tends to multiply at a fairly low rate and is present in the bloodstream in relatively low concentration. This strategy probably helps the virus avoid detection by the immune system's surveillance mechanism, which might lead to the virus being destroyed.

The virus does not appear to do much damage to the cells it infects, at least in the short term. The liver continues to function normally and the vast majority of persons infected have no specific symptoms to alert them to their liver infection. Over time, however, some of those infected will experience progressive damage to their livers, related to the effects of the virus on their hepatocytes and/or the effects of their immune systems attempting to eliminate the virus from the liver.

The liver has a tremendous potential to regenerate itself after damage, particularly if there is acute, self-limited damage or poisoning. However, in the case of a long-standing infection, liver cells can be lost and scarring or *fibrosis* can result. Fibrosis is the replacement of the original tissue with fibrous scar tissue. Fibrosis and liver-cell regeneration can be the precursor of liver cirrhosis. ("Cirrhosis" means that there is so much scar tissue that it completely surrounds areas of liver cells, isolating them from other liver cells.)

When liver damage is advanced, the liver may cease to perform its required functions and liver failure may ensue. Liver failure is eventually fatal unless the person has a liver transplant. Generally, however, liver failure does not happen until approximately 80 percent of the liver mass is lost. Cirrhosis can also be a risk factor for the development of liver cancer, as the frequent cycles of liver-cell injury and repair may result in alterations in the cells' genetic material that can predispose the liver to cancer.

It is generally only after many years or decades of infection that advanced liver disease occurs after hepatitis C virus infection. It is important to recognize that the majority of people infected with hepatitis C virus *will never have liver failure or liver cancer.*

# Other Organs of the Body

There is good evidence that hepatitis C virus infection can affect more than just the liver. In fact, it has been demonstrated that this virus can infect and perhaps multiply in the white blood cells of the body known as lymphocytes. Lymphocytes play a pivotal role in the body's immune defenses, making antibodies and battling infections and malignancies.

In some people chronically infected with hepatitis C virus, the lymphocytes are triggered to make abnormal antibodies that can react with the virus to form so-called immune complexes. These particular immune complexes may stick together when exposed to low temperature, so they are called *cryoglobulins* (*cryo* means cold; globulins are a form of protein). Cryoglobulins can cause a syndrome called *essential mixed cryoglobulinemia*, which can lead to arthritis, skin rashes, and nerve and kidney problems. Although cryoglobulins are frequently found in the blood of people infected with hepatitis C virus, only a very small minority of these people have any symptoms. The symptoms can run from mild to severe and life-threatening, although the latter is exceedingly uncommon. Successful treatment of hepatitis C virus can reverse the symptoms of essential mixed cryoglobulinemia.

## More about lymphocytes

Like all the other elements in the blood, lymphocytes start their life in bone marrow. However, lymphocytes are unique because they can circulate around the body and multiply in both the bloodstream and another circulatory system called the *lymphatic system*. In this system, lymphatic channels connect with lymph nodes (glands) located in the groin, armpits and neck; around the main blood vessels in the abdomen; near the bowels and in the chest. They are also directly connected to the liver and spleen. This gives the lymphocytes easy access to places where they are needed to fight invasions such as viral infections.

Hepatitis C infection can also show up through the development of *B-cell lymphoma*. Lymphoma is a cancer of the lymphocytes in the blood, lymph nodes, bone marrow and other organs. The B-lymphocytes affected are the ones involved in the production of antibodies. It is likely that B-cell lymphoma is related to cryoglobulinemia. Overall, it appears to be a rare occurrence in chronic hepatitis C infection. However, in some parts of the world—particularly Southern Europe—a substantial proportion of people with B-cell lymphomas test positive for hepatitis C.

There are other manifestations of hepatitis C virus outside the liver. A kidney disease known as *glomerulonephritis* is an inflammation that causes blood and protein in the urine, and may lead to permanent kidney damage. An uncommon skin condition called *lichen planus* features small, itchy, purplish-red patches that are often located on the fronts of the wrists and forearms, but may be found anywhere on the skin—even in the mouth or vagina or on the scalp. A condition involving the tear glands and salivary glands known as sicca syndrome causes dry mouth and eyes. Porphyria cutanea tarda, a blistering skin condition seen in a number of chronic liver diseases, affects the skin and nerves and is possibly related to an overload of iron. All of these *extrahepatic* (outside the liver) manifestations are uncommon. There also seems to be a higher than expected rate of diabetes in people infected with hepatitis C.

## Hepatitis C Virus and Other Viruses

Two other viruses that are commonly transmitted by exposure to blood are hepatitis B virus and the human immunodeficiency virus (HIV, the virus responsible for AIDS). In certain populations—for instance, people who had frequent exposure to blood and blood products prior to the availability of specific screening tests for these viruses, and people infected through intravenous drug use—two or even three of these viruses may be present at one time. The presence of multiple infections (known as *co-infection*) can modify the course and outcome of these infections.

Co-infection with both hepatitis C virus and hepatitis B virus can result in a worse outcome than either virus alone. Infection with both viruses increases the risk of liver cancer. These viruses can both be treated with interferon (discussed in Chapter 5), although the dose and duration of treatment are different. Typically, one virus is active while the other is dormant. Special tests can be done to determine which virus is active, and treatment can be tailored for that infection.

## Coinfection with Hepatitis C Virus and HIV Virus
Studies show that 50 to 90 percent of people infected with HIV are also infected with hepatitis C virus. Those with this co-infection progress to cirrhosis more rapidly. Treatment in this situation must be individualized, because there are few studies available to guide physicians. The effects of the viruses on each other, as well as the effects of drugs used for one virus on the other virus, and the interactions of the multiple drugs used, must all be considered.

# T W O

*Diagnosis and
Staging*

everal categories of blood tests are used in evaluating
people infected with hepatitis C virus. There are tests of
liver function and liver inflammation that are not specific to the virus. Additionally, there are tests that are specific
for hepatitis C virus. These can be further divided into tests
that detect antibodies against the virus and molecular assays
that detect and characterize the virus directly. However, the
most informative test for the staging and prognosis of hepatitis C remains the *liver biopsy*, discussed later in this chapter.

## Liver Enzymes

The liver *transaminases* (or liver enzymes) are alanine aminotransferase (ALT) and aspartate aminotransferase (AST)—
also called SGPT and SGOT, respectively. ALT and AST are
found in high concentration within liver cells, where they are
important in the manufacture of proteins. They are released
into the blood when liver cells are damaged. They are not at
all specific, and may be increased due to damage to other
organs such as heart, muscle, brain and kidney. Even within
the liver, there are many different potential causes for
increased liver enzymes. These include viral hepatitis, drug

reactions, alcohol, metabolic diseases and fat in the liver. The level of enzyme elevation says little about the cause or severity of the liver disease, and it is possible to have severe liver disease despite having persistently normal liver transaminases.

## True Liver Function Tests

Other blood tests can give insight into how the liver is actually functioning. The most sensitive of these is the *prothrombin time* (sometimes expressed as a ratio to normal, the International Normalized Ratio or INR), which is a measure of the time it takes blood to clot. Many of the blood factors involved in clotting are made in the liver, and if liver function is impaired, the prothrombin time can increase.

Another indicator of liver function is the concentration of albumin in the blood. Albumin is the major protein circulating in the blood, and it is made exclusively in the liver. Diminished liver function can result in a lower level of albumin in the blood.

Bilirubin, a product of the breakdown of red blood cells, is normally processed and excreted by the liver. The bilirubin level in the blood can increase if liver function is diminished and bilirubin processing is therefore impaired.

Since the results of these tests can all be influenced by factors other than liver disease, all the tests are usually done

### Monitoring cirrhosis

A comprehensive scoring system, known as the Child-Pugh score, combines the results of prothrombin time and albumin and bilirubin levels with two clinical factors—the presence or absence of free fluid in the abdomen (ascites) and mental confusion related to liver disease (encephalopathy)—to give an overall score that is helpful in monitoring patients with cirrhosis. However, since the liver is a large organ and a normal individual has more liver function than he or she requires, these tests and scores are of limited value and tend to be abnormal only after 70 to 80 percent of liver function has been lost.

at the same time, to give the best possible estimate of overall liver function.

# Diagnostic Tests Specific to Hepatitis C Virus

There are two classes of tests specific to hepatitis C: serological (antibody) tests and molecular tests. Almost anyone who becomes infected with hepatitis C virus will develop antibodies to the virus within several weeks. These antibodies are produced by the immune system, but they are generally ineffective or inadequate in eliminating the virus. In a minority of people, the immune response does eliminate the virus, but even then antibodies to the virus may persist in the blood. There are also situations where "false-positive" antibody results occur: natural antibodies can react (generally weakly) in the antibody test, giving a "positive" result even though the person has never been exposed to the virus. Thus, a positive result on a hepatitis C virus antibody test does not always mean that someone is infected with the virus, and a supplementary test is required to confirm infection. (Less than 10 percent of these tests give false-positive results.)

### Hepatitis C Antibody Test

The first-generation hepatitis C virus antibody test, the EIA-1 (enzyme immunoassay), was introduced in 1990. It measured antibodies to only one region of the virus and had low sensitivity (that is, it failed to detect the virus in some people) and low specificity (frequent false positives). This test was replaced in 1992 by the EIA-2 test, which measured antibodies to three regions of the virus, resulting in a substantial improvement in sensitivity and some improvement in specificity. A third-generation test, EIA-3, is now widely used and offers slight improvements.

The improved second-generation and third-generation EIA tests mean that the ability to detect hepatitis C virus antibodies is excellent. This in turn means that the risk of infection from blood transfusion in developed countries has been virtually eliminated. The rate of false-positive results remains a problem. For this reason, supplemental tests have been developed to confirm positive EIA results.

One of the supplemental tests used is the RIBA-2 (*recombinant immunoblot assay*). This test detects the same antibodies to the same three regions of the virus as the EIA-2 test, but in a different format where each antibody is detected independently. RIBA-2 tests are scored as positive if antibodies to two or more of the three regions of the virus are detected, and negative if no antibodies are detected. When antibodies to only one region of the virus are present, the test is considered indeterminate and further testing is required.

### Testing for the Actual Hepatitis C Virus

Sensitive molecular tests have been developed for the detection, quantification and genotyping of hepatitis C virus RNA (HCV RNA). (Qualitative tests determine whether the virus is present in the blood; quantitative tests measure the viral concentration or *viral load* in the blood.)

*Qualitative* hepatitis C virus testing is desirable before antiviral treatment is considered, because it is important to verify that the virus is present in the blood. In people with antibodies to the virus who have normal liver transaminases (ALT levels), it is also important to eliminate the possibility of a spontaneously resolved infection or a false-positive result, and this can be done by checking for HCV RNA by the most sensitive test—that is, a qualitative one. Similarly, this test is used during and at the end of treatment to see if the treatment has eradicated the virus.

The exact role of *quantitative* testing remains to be defined. Some studies show that patients with higher viral loads are less likely to benefit from treatment. However, this is by no means definite, and a high viral load should not by itself exclude someone from consideration for treatment. The amount of virus in the blood is *not* a measure of the extent of liver injury.

As mentioned above, there are multiple hepatitis C virus genotypes, and people infected with genotypes 2 and 3 may not require as long a course of treatment as those infected with genotype 1. Thus, genotyping may be of value when treatment is being considered. For more on this, see Chapter 5.

## What Is a Liver Biopsy?

A liver biopsy is a test that involves removing a small piece of the liver for analysis under the microscope or, occasionally, by other even more sensitive methods. Typically the liver core obtained in a biopsy weighs only 10 to 20 milligrams, but it contains information important for diagnosis, prognosis and treatment decisions. Most experts advocate liver biopsy of any patient for whom antiviral treatment is being considered, and for certain patients who are not candidates for treatment. A liver biopsy is the only way to accurately assess the stage of liver disease. It is possible for a liver biopsy of someone with elevated liver transaminase values to be near-normal or to show only mild damage, while the biopsy of someone with normal liver enzymes may (rarely) show advanced liver injury. The liver biopsy can also suggest the presence of conditions in the liver other than hepatitis C, and this can be important knowledge for the physician treating the patient. These conditions may include the effects of alcohol, drugs and medications, and the presence of iron overload and fat.

There are two ways by which a small piece of liver can be safely obtained for detailed examination under the microscope: *percutaneous biopsy* and *transjugular biopsy*.

## Percutaneous Biopsy

This is the method used if you have normal blood clotting and no abnormal fluid in your abdomen. Your blood must be tested for its ability to clot, and it is important that for eight days prior to this test (and for a couple of days after the biopsy) no ASA products or arthritis pills called NSAIDs be taken, because they impair your blood's ability to clot.

On the day of the test you will arrive at the hospital early in the morning, because after the biopsy you have to lie flat or on your side in bed and have regular monitoring of your pulse and blood pressure for four to six hours. This means that almost your whole day will be spent at the hospital.

Some physicians give a short-acting sedative and painkiller just prior to the biopsy, to reduce any anxiety and potential discomfort. Once the best site for inserting the liver biopsy needle has been located, low down the ribcage on the right side, the area is frozen with a local anesthetic. Then a hollow needle is rapidly inserted into the liver capsule and a small amount of tissue is drawn up into the needle, which is removed from the liver in a matter of a few seconds.

### Possible Complications of Liver Biopsy

The reason you need to stay flat or on your side for four to six hours is that there is always a little bleeding when the biopsy needle pierces the capsule of the liver. Very rarely is the bleeding serious enough to require a blood transfusion (1 in 1,000 cases), although sometimes there is a small trickle of blood that will irritate the diaphragm and cause pain in the tip of the shoulder. (This is because the same nerve is associated with the diaphragm and the tip of the shoulder.) Now that the transjugular biopsy can be used for people whose blood does not clot normally, the risk of death from percutaneous biopsy is extraordinarily low.

Another complication is that the biopsy needle may pierce the gallbladder (which is just under the liver) rather than the liver. This is also very rare but, because it is a possibility, a few doctors choose to have liver biopsies done under ultrasound guidance. If the gallbladder is perforated, sudden, very severe pain in the abdomen develops immediately after the procedure, and it may be necessary to operate to remove the damaged gallbladder.

### Transjugular Biopsy

Transjugular biopsy is used if your blood clotting is impaired (meaning that the risk of bleeding from a pierced liver capsule is too high), for example, when the patient has ascites (fluid in the abdomen). The liver capsule is very unlikely to be pierced using the transjugular method.

After injection of local anesthetic to numb the area, a small cut is made in the right side of the neck. Since transjugular biopsy has to be done under X-ray guidance, the physician conducting the test is generally a radiologist. He or she will introduce a sterile, long, thin tube into the vein in the neck. The tube is then passed through natural openings in the heart, through to the veins draining the liver. Once the tube is in the liver, a very long biopsy needle is passed through the tube into the middle of the liver, where a piece of liver tissue is taken.

If there is bleeding from the liver after a transjugular biopsy, the blood will flow directly into the liver's own vein. In other words, there is no leakage of blood from the liver.

Because it is a little frightening to be lying on an X-ray table for 30 minutes or more, sedation is always given. The same monitoring of the blood pressure and pulse are required following this test to make sure no unusual bleeding has occurred.

## After the Biopsy

Following either method of liver biopsy, there may be some discomfort in the upper right side of your abdomen or in your right shoulder. This should not be severe and requires no treatment. You can return to work and resume all other usual activities the following day. It is probably advisable to avoid any trips out of town for the next week because, occasionally, bleeding occurs up to four days after a liver biopsy. If you have any symptoms of dizziness, fainting spells or severe abdominal pain, call your physician's office and go to the emergency room at once. You need immediate attention.

## Interpretation of the Liver Biopsy

The pathologist reviewing the liver biopsy is assessing it with respect to two main factors: inflammation and fibrosis (scarring). Under one grading system, inflammation is scored from grade 0 (normal) to 4 and fibrosis is graded from stage 0 to 4, with stage 4 being cirrhosis. There are other grading systems used—the hepatitis activity index (HAI), more commonly used in the U.S.A., employs a larger scale of 22 points—but essentially they all mean the same thing. The grade of inflammation represents the immune system's activity against the virus at the time of the biopsy. Inflammation leads to damage of hepatocytes that repair themselves by regeneration and/or scarring or fibrosis. The fibrosis grade can be thought of as the cumulative effect of all the inflammation that has gone on since the time of infection.

Fibrosis of the liver is a precursor of cirrhosis, and the finding of *strands* of fibrosis is the best predictor of the potential for later development of cirrhosis (*circles* of fibrosis). As such, it is an important factor in the decision to treat or not to treat. Since the disease progresses over years or even decades, this information must be interpreted in the context of duration of infection (if it is known) and the person's age and life expectancy. In cases where antiviral treatment is not started, it may be appropriate to repeat the liver biopsy after three to five years, to estimate the rate of progression of the disease.

# T H R E E

## *What's Next?*

If you have just discovered that you have hepatitis C, you may be handling the challenges well, or you may feel overwhelmed by them. In either case, it is a difficult, demanding situation, and you may need help. First, you need to deal with the emotional impact of being told that you have a potentially lifelong chronic disease. Once you overcome this stage, you will be ready to seek support and to investigate the facts about the disease. Having strong support from others and knowing all the facts about your hepatitis C, you will be able to deal with the disease more effectively, protect your liver from unnecessary damage and thus prolong your life. The sooner you are able to start dealing with your hepatitis C, the better you will feel about yourself. The tips in this chapter may help you in this adjustment.

## Handling the Diagnosis

Valerie, age 55, had never been sick before in her life, so she was devastated when she tested positive for hepatitis C, in a blood test taken when she applied for life insurance. She did not want to tell her family that she had hepatitis C, because she was afraid that her husband might think she had cheated on him, and that she might lose the respect of her children. She decided not to let her family know, and she tried to deal with the problem by herself. Fearing that she might give the virus to her grandchildren, she made up all kinds of excuses to stay away from them.

After a year of keeping the diagnosis to herself, Valerie had become isolated and depressed. What made her even more upset was that she could not consider any treatment, because she was afraid her family and friends might find out about her disease. She eventually discussed her problem, one year later, when she came to her family doctor's clinic in tears and admitted how lonely and miserable she felt, and said she had plans to commit suicide.

In Valerie's case, the greatest health risk was not the hepatitis C but the extreme anxiety and depression she felt from dealing with her diagnosis on her own. Once she learned about routes of transmission of the hepatitis C virus, she realized that she must have been infected when she was a little girl, by a needle reused for vaccination; she had had this infection for most of her life. With the encouragement of her hepatitis healthcare team, she eventually felt comfortable about letting her family know of her diagnosis. Every time she came into the clinic, she brought in a different family member to discuss his or her questions or concerns. It took a lot of effort for her to tell the first family member the news, but the revelation got easier with time. With the support of her family, Valerie is now thinking about starting treatment.

**Initial Reaction**
It is normal to feel sorry for yourself in the beginning, but this emotion, if allowed to persist, can cause a constant drain of energy. If you believe that all the potential complications of hepatitis C, including an early death, are coming your way soon, you are sure to feel anxious and fearful, and you may

**Dealing with the diagnosis**
- Resolve your anxiety.
- Seek strong support.
- Educate yourself about the disorder.
- Learn the facts about hepatitis C transmission.

feel depressed. Alternatively, you may suppress your feelings and just live for the moment, ignoring the precautions that could improve your odds. When you believe nothing will do any good, you may do little or nothing to improve the status of your hepatitis C.

**Positive Steps**

When you start to realize that you can reduce the risk of complications and thus early death, you will become more hopeful. You may still be anxious, but your anxiety can be resolved if you understand clearly the problems you face, and the treatments and supportive measures that can be taken, and have a reasonable and realistic estimate of the discomfort or inconvenience you can expect. Hence, it is important to learn about the physiology and complications of hepatitis C, and the treatments and other protective measures required to lessen the severity of your disease.

When you have overcome your initial anxiety by learning the facts about hepatitis C, you should be sufficiently relaxed to follow instructions better, and to do the right things to help your liver and hence yourself. Therefore, any energy spent on negative feelings should be redirected into positive actions for a better outcome.

When you first learn that you have hepatitis C, it can help to find strong support to assist you in dealing with your emotional issues. You can call upon relatives, friends, other people with hepatitis C or professionals dealing with the disease to back you up, but only if you feel comfortable having them participate in your healthcare. By talking to your spouse or a best friend, you may be able to share some of your anxiety, and feel more at ease.

It is best to talk to a friend who has some knowledge of hepatitis C, because the disease is complicated and some people are unnecessarily scared of becoming infected too. You may be shocked to find people treating you differently after you tell them about your illness. Some may think of hepatitis C as a killer disease. Others may be afraid of catching hepatitis C infection just from being near you. So before you go telling everyone the news, think about which people will be supportive. If you think a certain person will not be, don't say anything.

Is it less of a headache not to tell anyone, but just keep the news to yourself? Only you can answer this question. Your decision should depend on the trust in the relationship between you and the people you intend to tell. Remember, though, that additional stress can arise if you feel guilty not sharing the news with your family members or the people you are living with. After all, you hope they trust you and like you for who you are, and the fact that you have hepatitis C should not change that.

You may have to educate your relatives or friends about hepatitis C. Many people get the different forms of hepatitis mixed up. As well, hepatitis C affects some people more severely than others, and therefore the problems one individual encounters are very different from those of another. Your hepatitis C condition may not be at all the same as that of other people your family, friends or support group have come in contact with. Clarify the situation by making sure your family and friends understand the nature of *your* problem, and *your* requirements for treatment. Give them this book to read.

## Myths and misconceptions about hepatitis C

- that hepatitis C virus can be transmitted through casual contact such as shaking hands, talking and drinking from the same cup
- that people with hepatitis C should separate their eating utensils from others'
- that hepatitis C virus is less easily transmitted than HIV
- that hepatitis C virus infection is less deadly than HIV infection
- that there is a vaccine for hepatitis C
- that hepatitis C virus means intravenous drug abuse
- that those with hepatitis C should not use public facilities such as swimming pools

You not only have to deal with your emotional issues at this stage; you also have to deal with others' concerns. It is not easy to handle all these issues, but you have to participate in the process to make you feel better about living with your disease. Be ready to give people the facts about hepatitis C and, more specifically, about your case, so they can feel more comfortable being around you and helping you. They may not ask you directly, because they are afraid of hurting your feelings, but people usually wonder how you came in contact with this infection, and whether or not they will catch it from you. You need to know the facts about hepatitis C transmission, to educate your family and friends and to ease their fear of getting the disease from you.

## How Is Hepatitis C Spread?

### Blood Products
The virus circulates in the blood, so it can only be transmitted by blood-to-blood contact. Prior to mid-1990, people who received a transfusion of blood or blood products were at risk of coming in contact with hepatitis C, because there was

no specific test for the virus. Since May 1990, blood donated in North America has been screened for the antibody to the hepatitis C virus before it is put into the blood supply. These days, blood donated in Canada and in most places in the U.S.A. is tested for the actual virus, HCV RNA, not just for the antibody, before the blood is put into the blood supply. Thus the risk of acquiring hepatitis C now from a transfusion in North America should be close to zero. Unfortunately, this is not the case worldwide. The rate of people contracting hepatitis C virus via blood transfusion is high in developing countries where hepatitis C screening is not conducted.

### Contaminated Needles or Other Equipment

One of the most common ways by which hepatitis C is spread today is through the use of injected drugs, when people share syringes, needles and/or other equipment. Sharing only has to occur once for the virus to spread. "Snorting" cocaine using the same straw as a person infected with hepatitis C is another known risk factor for acquiring an infection. Furthermore, it is possible to transmit the virus via contaminated needles used in body piercing or tattooing. Some people with hepatitis C who have come from developing countries likely got their infection from poorly sterilized needles used for injection and/or vaccination many years ago. It is possible to have hepatitis for fifty or sixty years and not know it!

---

### Transmission of hepatitis C
Prior to 1990, hepatitis C was sometimes transmitted through blood transfusion. These days, in North America, it is most commonly spread **through the use of contaminated needles or other equipment.**
    Less often it is passed from mother to infant at birth, and it may possibly be spread during sexual contact or within a household.

Medical care obtained anywhere before the advent of disposable needles and syringes represented a risk for contracting hepatitis C. In some areas of the world, tattooing, body piercing, circumcision (male and female) and surgery continue to be performed in a way that allows the transmission of hepatitis C.

## Sexual Transmission

Hepatitis C virus is not detectable in saliva or semen unless the sample is contaminated with blood, but a very small percentage of people do become infected via sexual contact. The disease could be transmitted from a woman to her partner if they have intercourse when the woman has her menstrual period, if there is a sore with a break in the skin on the sexual organs of her partner that will allow the transfer of the infected menstrual blood. However, when sexual transmission is thought to have taken place, it is more likely to have spread from male to female. The hepatitis C infection rate is higher among people who are sexually active with several partners, especially those with a history of a sexually transmitted disease. (Genital herpes is quite common, and many people forget that it is a sexually transmitted disease.) If you kiss a person on the mouth and both of you have open sores and/or bleeding gums, it is possible, although very unlikely, that hepatitis C could be transmitted. The virus can also be transmitted when no precaution is taken during traumatic sexual intercourse (i.e., intercourse that causes bleeding, even in minute amounts), by exposure to blood-tinged saliva or through other forms of intimate blood-to-blood contact with an infected person. If both sexual partners are infected with the virus, it is not uncommon that each obtained the infection independently, through one or another form of risky behavior.

**Transmission from Mother to Infant (Vertical Spread)**
Although the hepatitis C virus RNA and the antibody can be detected in the blood of an infant born to a hepatitis C carrier for up to one year after birth, studies done in such babies have found that they rarely contract the disease permanently. The rate at which they do is about 6 to 7 percent. Long-term spread from mother to infant is more likely when high levels of the virus are present in the mother's blood. The infant has a higher risk of contracting hepatitis C—15 to 20 percent—if the mother is also infected with HIV. There are no cases reported where a nursing child has been infected with hepatitis C through breast milk, so women with chronic hepatitis C should not be discouraged from breastfeeding. However, it's important for the mother to be comfortable with this decision.

**Transmission within the Household (Horizontal Spread)**
So far, there has not been any evidence that the hepatitis C virus spreads among people in the household except via sexual activity. The hepatitis C virus is *not* present in most body secretions, including semen, urine and saliva, unless they contain blood particles. So it is safe to kiss, hug or hold hands with your family members or friends. Furthermore, it is not appropriate or necessary to use separate bathroom facilities or eating utensils, such as cups, bowls, cutlery and so on. Others will not get hepatitis C from eating food prepared by you. But it is wise that you not share items such as razor blades and toothbrushes, which may have been in contact with traces of blood.

**Unknown Source**
About 10 percent of people who have been infected with hepatitis C infection cannot recall any factors that may have put them at risk. Some may have forgotten that they used an injected drug

just once or twice at a party as a teenager; others may have received injections as a child with non-disposable needles, or had blood transfusions they knew nothing about during surgery.

**Learning More about Transmission**
If you want to know more about hepatitis C, talk to your physician or other members of your hepatitis C healthcare team. You should be cautious about statements made by friends, relatives and acquaintances, or claims reported in the media (over television and radio, in newspapers or magazines or over the Internet) because the information may be incorrect. Remember, bad news sells well and travels fast! You may want to verify any up-to-date news on the disease with your doctor or nurse, to gain a better understanding of what you are reading.

Your family and friends may want to be included in your medical consultations, so that they can become part of your informed support team. This will also give them a chance to ask questions about concerns they may have. Many of the misconceptions about hepatitis C stem from miscommunication or misinformation from the family or a close friend who has heard about a "cure" somewhere, or about someone who has had "better" treatment. It is very easy to feel overloaded when so much information is being thrown at you from your family, friends, the media and doctors and nurses. Remember, you cannot take in everything at once. Set priorities. By making sure that all interested parties are kept informed, you can all focus your energy and efforts along the most constructive channel.

## Preventing the Spread
Because no vaccine is available for hepatitis C at this time, take care in dealing with any blood products or blood-contaminated items. You may want to consider the facts and suggestions listed below, to protect others and prevent the spread of the virus.

- You are not allowed to donate your blood or your organs (the latter may be allowed in rare instances).
- Dispose of blood-soaked materials yourself, rather than pass the task on to others.
- Clean up blood spills with household bleach (5 percent solution).
- If you use needles and syringes for whatever purpose, discard them immediately. Never reuse them. They are usually placed inside a "sharps" container or glass jar that is disposed of only at a healthcare institution.
- Avoid body piercing and tattoos.
- Never share "straws" for cocaine use.
- Because the virus is hard to kill and can exist in almost invisible amounts of blood, do not share personal items that may be contaminated by blood, such as razors, tweezers, nail-clippers, scissors or toothbrushes. It is not known how long the virus can remain alive outside the body, but it makes sense to avoid sharing these items.
- Keep latex or rubber gloves handy in case blood contact is unavoidable—in a first aid emergency, for example. Ask a healthcare professional to demonstrate the safe removal of soiled gloves.
- The rate of transmission by sexual contact is considered so low that condoms are not recommended in a mutually monogamous relationship. However, the virus may be transmitted via genital herpes virus and other sexually transmitted diseases. Therefore, it is important to use condoms when you have any genital lesions or if you have multiple sexual partners.
- Since hepatitis C has been found in menstrual blood, and because it is theoretically possible to infect your partner during sex, women with hepatitis C virus should either avoid sex during menstruation or practice only safe sex at these times.

- You should inform your dentist and other healthcare professionals that you test positive for hepatitis C. They should be practicing "universal precautions" anyway, but your statement will help to ensure this.

## Seeking Support

Once you have absorbed the details of your diagnosis and have learned more about hepatitis C, seek further information from your healthcare providers about the stage of your disease and the treatment options that are available to you.

You may wonder why you might need treatment right now, if you have few or no symptoms. Indeed, this symptom-free stage makes it difficult for many people to believe they really have hepatitis C. But there are things you can do early in the infection that lessen the chance of it causing severe disease. Do not wait until you have developed symptoms of liver failure before seeking advice.

Although there is so far no treatment for hepatitis C that offers a 100-percent guaranteed cure, the chance of stopping the virus from multiplying or slowing down the damage is rapidly improving with today's treatment regimens. However, not everyone with hepatitis C infection needs treatment; it depends on the severity of the liver damage. Chapter 5 will cover in detail the treatments currently available and their side effects. You may also want to consider the factors listed in Chapter 7, "What Can I Do to Help Myself?"

Talk to your physician or nurse about your needs, concerns, questions and problems. Remember that you are the focus. The healthcare team's goal is to help you to understand as much as possible about your hepatitis C, to offer you the treatment options available for you and to help you to live with the disease. Speak up when you do not understand something you are told. Also indicate when too much information is being given to you. Perhaps you can arrange another appointment for a later date.

If you do not feel that you are receiving enough support from the healthcare staff and your family and close friends, you may want to participate in a hepatitis support group. Besides gaining the companionship of people with the same chronic infection, you will have the opportunity to talk about any problem or concern you have, whether it is related to your hepatitis C or not. In addition, knowing that there are other people out there with the same problem will make you feel less isolated and lonely, which in turn can lift your spirits and reduce your anxiety. However, it is important to talk only to people who have a positive outlook on life in general as well as on their chronic hepatitis C. You need support, not discouragement! If you encounter people who only like to complain or tell horror stories, stay away from them. Select a support group in which people emphasize abilities rather than disabilities, and solutions rather than problems. Of course, you may describe the difficulties you are experiencing, but you should be encouraged to overcome these difficulties. In other words, don't become a victim of the disease.

## Stages of Grieving

The natural stages of grieving apply not only to bereavement but to other losses in life. An understanding of these natural stages can assist you to understand your feelings when you have just learned about your hepatitis C diagnosis. These stages also come into play as you learn to cope in the future.

Sister Calista Roy, a nursing theorist, described the four major stages of coping with a loss as follows:
1. shock and denial
2. understanding the loss
3. attempting to deal with the loss
4. final resolution

It is certainly a health loss when people are diagnosed with a chronic hepatitis C infection. Not everyone will demonstrate all of the behaviors discussed below, but each grieving person will show some of the behaviors described.

*Dealing with Shock and Denial*
How you react to the diagnosis of hepatitis C depends on your personality and how you usually cope with and adapt to life's problems. This stage may last a few minutes to days. If you are a person who regards bad luck as just one more problem to be handled with determination, or as something you simply have to make the best of, this positive attitude will probably carry you through the initial shock of the diagnosis. However, if you usually react to bad luck by asking, "Why me?" you may spend most of your emotional energy being angry at the disease, the "gods" or other people for bringing this misery down on you! Anger is a normal reaction, and in some ways it can help you through the period of grieving that takes place immediately after the diagnosis is made. You may refuse to accept the diagnosis altogether: "Oh no, it can't be true." It is normal to react this way but the fact is, you have hepatitis C infection, and you need to learn how to manage it right now. It is important to apply angry energy in a positive and useful direction.

Robbie, who is 61 years old and was divorced five years ago, was very upset at the news that she has hepatitis C. She had no risk factors. She did not use intravenous drugs, she had not had tattoos or blood transfusions and she had had only one sexual partner, her ex-husband. She strongly believed that her husband had cheated on her, and that that was how she had caught this disease. She was very angry at her ex-husband for giving her the disease, so she decided to take one week of vacation to look for him, to find out for sure whether he was responsible. Yet she was so certain in her heart that he had infected her that she excluded all other possible risk factors. Was it worthwhile spending vacation time and money to find out whether he was really to blame? She might have contracted her hepatitis C by sharing toothbrushes with her friends in boarding school, or from the reused vaccination needles she remembered from when she was a child.

The healthcare team has advised Robbie to accept the fact that she has hepatitis C today, and to do all she can to prevent any further liver damage, rather than spend her energy on a past that cannot be changed.

## Understanding the Disease

It may not be easy to accept the fact that you have hepatitis C but, with time, the reality of your diagnosis will become believable. At this stage you become interested in learning more about the disease. You may start with questions like:

- What is hepatitis C?
- How did I get it?
- Will my family members or friends get it from me?
- How can hepatitis C affect me?
- Is there anything I can do right now to prolong my life?

If you are interested in obtaining answers to these questions, you are ready to move on to the next stage in dealing with the diagnosis. Remember, this stage takes a lot of time and energy, as you gather information from different sources and put it all together so that it makes sense. So take your time!

You may be able to figure out how you acquired this disease. Unfortunately, 10 percent or more of people with hepatitis C do not know where or when they acquired it. You may feel unnecessarily guilty if you exposed yourself to the infection due to foolish or immature behavior many years ago. You may feel angry if you believe someone else is responsible for your being infected. This is a normal reaction. Now it is important for you to learn how to deal with the situation.

*Attempting to Deal with the Disease*
The appropriate support network and information from your physician will help you learn about the types of treatment available, what advantages and disadvantages each treatment has and what kind of financial or psychological support groups are out there in the community for you (see Further Resources, at the end of this book). After obtaining all the information, you should develop a positive approach to helping yourself. Currently, the treatment options for hepatitis C are different types of interferon and Rebetron (a combination of interferon alpha 2b and ribavirin). The treatment is expensive and the treatment duration is long. It is important to find out all available resources before you are encumbered with this big expense in time and money. There are very few people who can afford to pay for treatment themselves. The doctor or nurse who is in charge of your case should know about the resources available, so that you can obtain treatment with the least expense or even at no cost to you. The situation depends on your medical coverage and your financial situation.

You should also discuss the side effects that you can expect from treatment with interferon and ribavirin. There is no type of drug treatment that does not have side effects. Dealing with these side effects is covered in Chapter 5.

*Final Resolution*
There are still more failures than successes in our treatments for hepatitis C. About 60 percent of those treated do not respond, while about 40 percent do. The reason for this difference in response is explained in Chapter 5.

You may find out that you have not responded to the treatment as early as 12 or 24 weeks into treatment. If you lose the virus during treatment, there is a 50 percent to 75 percent chance that it will remain inactive once treatment is discontinued. Unfortunately, the virus may return. Relapses occur in about 25 percent or more patients after the treatment is stopped. But even if the virus returns after the treatment stops, the treatment will have made the virus inactive for a while. At least the liver had a break from the virus during the treatment period. There is some recent evidence that interferon therapy benefits the liver and may reduce the rate of liver cancer, even in those who are "non-responders."

If the treatment eradicates the virus for six months, the news is good. You have a 95 percent chance of staying virus-free. For how long? We don't know for sure, as followup studies have so far produced data for only up to ten years, but it is anticipated that the virus will not return. Studies also show that liver damage stops and there is a gradual improvement in those who have permanently lost detectable HCV RNA from their blood after completing treatment.

# F O U R

# Symptoms

## At the Time of Initial Infection

When you first contract the virus, you will likely notice nothing. In fact, only one-third of people infected with hepatitis C actually feel ill, with flu-like symptoms such as nausea and vomiting, upset stomach, low fever, tiredness, muscle aches and loss of appetite. There is a 10 percent chance that you will have yellowing of the whites of the eyes and skin (jaundice) and dark urine. The flu-like symptoms generally go away within two to twelve weeks. However, in some people, tiredness persists for a while longer. Most often the diagnosis of hepatitis C is missed at the time of the initial infection, because there are no symptoms and hence the appropriate blood tests are not done to identify the infection.

## Once the Hepatitis C Is Chronic

Less than 50 percent of those infected with hepatitis C are able to get rid of the virus and clear their infection on their own. The rest carry the virus infection in their body for many, many years, but most have no symptoms. By medical definition, you become a "chronic carrier" of this virus when it persists in your body for more than six months. It is not unusual for someone who feels absolutely well to have serious disease and, conversely, those who have severe symptoms may have

## Some general symptoms of hepatitis C infection

- tiredness
- abdominal discomfort
- nausea
- poor appetite
- sleep disturbance
- itching
- depression

only mild liver disease. As well, the course of the liver disease is different in each individual.

Joe found out that he had chronic hepatitis C virus infection at the time he applied for his life insurance. The diagnosis was a shock to him because he had felt healthy all his life. He had no idea how he had contracted the virus and he could not recall any major illnesses.

Nancy went for her annual medical checkup only to find out that her liver enzymes were high. Her family physician investigated further, with more blood tests, and found that she tested positive for the antibody to hepatitis C (HCV Ab). Nancy could remember one episode of a "very bad" flu-like feeling about six months earlier. She recalled feeling nauseated, with some associated vomiting and stomach pains. She had also noticed that her urine was very dark at that time. She had not sought medical attention, however, and had recovered three weeks later.

John was diagnosed with chronic hepatitis over twenty years ago. It was initially called non-A, non-B hepatitis, and later diagnosed as hepatitis C. The cause of his infection was most likely his intravenous drug use as a teenager. Although the virus has been present all these years, John has felt fine except for some tiredness and an occasional dull pain on the right side of his belly. Nothing has been sufficiently troublesome to interfere with his life, with a full-time job and a wife and two children.

The symptoms John experienced are not specific to hepatitis C infection, in that they can be experienced by many individuals, some who are otherwise quite well, and others who have different types of chronic diseases, such as multiple sclerosis or systemic lupus erythematosus.

## Some Commonly Reported Symptoms

### Tiredness

Tiredness is very common among people with any type of chronic illness. They describe it as lack of energy and stamina, a feeling of weakness, a malaise and sluggishness. As the feeling of fatigue is a very personal and subjective complaint, your definition and interpretation of tiredness may be different from that of others with hepatitis C.

Amanda is a 42-year-old housewife who has been feeling tired for the past ten years. She describes her tiredness as "dead tired," "no energy," "total body exhaustion" and feeling as if "her whole body has been punched." Her tiredness is not relieved by a good night's sleep. Indeed, she finds the more she sleeps, the more tired she feels. She was recently diagnosed with chronic hepatitis C, and she decided to seek counseling.

Amanda has learned to organize her activities and to prioritize her household chores at the beginning of each day. She does not attempt more than one heavy-duty activity in a day. For example, she vacuums on Monday and leaves the laundry for Tuesday. She has also started a low-impact aerobics class three times a week. She continues to take her afternoon nap, which she finds necessary. She still feels tired, but she realizes that she can accomplish more by organizing her day so that she feels good about herself, and this has helped to distract her from focusing on her tiredness.

In extreme, rare situations, tiredness can be so debilitating that the person becomes totally dependent on others to carry out normal daily activities. It is logical to think that the more tired you feel, the more severe your liver disease must be. However, this is not so. There are many as-yet-unproven explanations for this phenomenon.

In the last few years, experts have become more aware of the impact of hepatitis C infection on a person's well-being. This well-being can be measured by means of a quality-of-life assessment. Several studies have shown that people with chronic hepatitis C infection have poor quality-of-life scores in areas that measure bodily symptoms—that is, energy level, fatigue and pain. One study indicated that those who had previously used intravenous drugs felt more tired than those who had not used drugs. This is not surprising, because narcotics alter the brain receptors for pain and associated symptoms.

## Abdominal Discomfort

Abdominal discomfort is commonly reported by people infected with hepatitis C. It may be just a dull ache along the lower edge of the liver, located on the right upper side of the abdomen. Hence, it is often referred to as "right upper quadrant pain." Other people say that the pain can sometimes be severe but is not long-lasting. Most say that they do not feel actual pain but that it is a nuisance to feel "something" aching that comes and goes in the abdomen.

Some experts believe that this symptom has little to do with the liver disease, because the liver is not well supplied with nerve fibers. Others suspect that these aches and discomforts are due to inflammation of the lining of the liver. In fact, this inflammation of the outer lining of the liver may be seen when the liver is examined at the time of a liver transplant. If pain is present, this should be brought to your doctor's attention to exclude other possible causes such as gallstones.

### Nausea

You may feel nauseated at the same time that you experience the abdominal discomfort. This feeling of nausea is generally mild and is not restricted to a particular time of the day. There is usually no associated vomiting. Medication is seldom required for this symptom but, again, it is annoying to feel intermittent nausea throughout the day. In more serious cases, an anti-nausea drug such as dimenhydrinate may help to relieve this symptom. However, dimenhydrinate can cause sleepiness so you should not use it if you are driving a vehicle.

### Poor Appetite

Losing your appetite is also common. However, it is important not to develop the habit of skipping meals, being a picky eater and relying on vitamin supplements rather than getting your nutrition from natural sources. This lack of appetite, which is generally due to a combination of factors such as tiredness, depression, pain and lack of sleep, occasionally causes weight loss. If you have severe nausea, you should try eating small, frequent meals instead of three regular meals a day. Adding different herbs and spices in cooking also helps to stimulate your taste buds. Exercise is another good way to increase the appetite.

### Sleep Disturbance

Sleep disturbance includes both having trouble falling asleep at night and waking up many times during normal sleeping hours. This will obviously cause you to feel unrefreshed on getting up in the morning. Your sleeping pattern may completely reverse—

you sleep during the day and are awake at night. (This generally only happens when you have severe liver disease, that is, liver failure.) Very often, sleeping pills are prescribed for this problem. Taking sleeping pills is not a good practice to get into, as most are very addictive. Improving your sleep regimen should be the first step. Reading or having a warm drink before you go to bed may help. Avoid stimulants such as tea, coffee, smoking or excessive exercise for several hours before going to bed. Taking sleeping pills should be your last resort. If your doctor does prescribe sleeping pills, make sure that they are not benzodiazepines, such as lorazepam, diazepam and oxazepam. These should be avoided by anyone who has severe liver disease.

### Itching

Itchiness can be either confined to certain parts of the body—for example, both legs—or all over the body. Generally there is no skin rash. The exact cause of itching is not known. You may find your itchiness gets worse in winter months when your skin and the inside air are drier. When the itchiness is mild and intermittent, antihistamines will help, but avoid those that make you drowsy. In most situations all that is needed for your dry skin is baby oil in your bathwater, or a good emollient lotion. Sometimes you may scratch yourself during your sleep, so that when you awaken your body is covered with scratch marks. In this case, cut your fingernails short and wear thin gloves in bed, to reduce surface damage to the skin. If such severe itching persists, consult your physician for medication to relieve the symptom.

### Depression

Being given a diagnosis of chronic hepatitis C is a depressing experience in itself. It is most likely that you will get over your initial depression and carry on with your normal life, but some people remain depressed for an extended period of time.

One study has shown that depressive disorders are a major reason why some people with hepatitis C have trouble coping with day-to-day activities. It is wise to seek professional help when you feel depressed, before the feeling becomes so severe that you want to harm yourself.

Depression is very common in our society. There is no shame in seeing a psychologist or a psychiatrist who will support you and give you treatment if necessary. Antidepressant drugs are often helpful, and are safe to take even if you have liver disease. Signs of depression often go along with other physical symptoms such as lack of motivation, tiredness, loss of appetite and inability to sleep. When the depression is successfully treated, these other symptoms generally improve as well.

## Less Common Symptoms
The following symptoms appear less often.

- dry eyes and mouth (sicca syndrome)
- ulcer of the eye (Mooren's corneal ulcer)
- muscle and joint aches
- dizziness
- decreased memory
- decreased concentration
- rash (red blotches, most often on legs)
- blistering skin lesions

Remember that these symptoms can be experienced by people who do not have hepatitis C. It is best to discuss your symptoms with healthcare professionals, so they can help you learn ways to manage the symptoms successfully.

## What Is Going to Happen to Me?
As the virus attacks the liver, liver cells die. Fortunately, when liver cells die, they are replaced by new ones. But if the inflam-

mation caused by the virus is severe enough, it may lead to development of scar tissue (fibrosis). As more scar tissue develops, the liver becomes hardened. The term "cirrhosis" refers to the stage when the scarring surrounds clumps of liver cells. A cirrhotic liver is lumpy and hard. Whether you have cirrhosis or not cannot always be confirmed by a simple test such as an ultrasound examination. A liver biopsy is more precise.

The changes in the structure of the liver prevent the blood from flowing smoothly through the liver. As a result, blood often bypasses the clumps of liver cells surrounded by scar tissue. This means that there is a reduced blood supply to these liver cells, and so the functioning of the liver is reduced over time.

Whether or not your liver will progress through all the stages of fibrosis to full-blown cirrhosis is hard to predict. In most people infected with hepatitis C, little damage to the liver is observed for the first 20 to 40 years following infection. But some people progress to a more advanced stage sooner.

There are now a number of studies reporting on the outcome of hepatitis C infection, from contaminated blood products, in children and young women. These indicate that cirrhosis is found in 2 to 8 percent twenty years after the initial infection. Other studies have examined different patient populations—for example, those infected similarly but when older. It seems that hepatitis C causes a more rapidly progressing disease when it is acquired after the age of forty.

## Factors That Promote Severe Disease
There are some well-known risk factors that promote more rapid progression of the disease. Your liver disease will get worse faster if you

- are male
- were first infected after the age of forty
- have a fat abdomen

- consume more than two to three drinks of alcohol every day
- are also infected with the AIDS virus
- use medications that depress the immune system—for example, anticancer drugs, steroids or anti-rejection drugs (taken by people after an organ transplant)

If your liver enzyme (ALT) levels are persistently normal, you have a smaller chance of developing cirrhosis than someone who has persistently abnormal ALT levels. Even if you have developed cirrhosis, the chance of there being further deterioration over the next ten years is 25 to 50 percent.

## What Happens in Cirrhosis?

Cirrhosis is characterized by three features: liver-cell regeneration, clumps of cells (*nodules*) in the liver and fibrosis. Contrary to popular belief, cirrhosis is not caused exclusively by alcohol.

In the early stages, the liver can compensate for cirrhosis. There remains a sufficient mass of liver cells to perform the functions of the organ, so bilirubin, albumin and blood-clotting tests can all be normal. With more advanced cirrhosis, these tests may become abnormal. Additionally, cirrhosis is a risk factor in the development of liver cancer.

### Cirrhosis and liver complications

A large study in France followed 416 patients with cirrhosis due to infection with hepatitis C. When these patients first entered the study, they had no evidence of liver decompensation. They were followed for up to ten years. Liver cancer developed in 60 of these people and, overall, 83 died in the followup period (including 34 with liver cancer). Almost all the deaths were related to liver disease. The risk of dying within five years was 15.3 percent. Patients who had low albumin levels in their blood had the highest risk of dying. Reports from Italy and the U.S.A. have shown similar results.

**Complications**

Cirrhosis may be associated with few or no symptoms at an early stage. The complications of cirrhosis include:

- yellowing of eyes and skin
- abdominal swelling and ankle swelling
- increased blood pressure in the portal vein
- internal bleeding from large veins in the esophagus and stomach
- personality changes and mental confusion
- easy bruising

If any of these events take place, the liver is said to have "decompensated," meaning that there are not enough healthy cells left to allow the liver to function. Liver transplantation must then be considered.

### Yellowing of Eyes and Skin (Jaundice)

Jaundice is often a sign of a deteriorating liver. The yellowness seen in the whites of the eyes and skin is due to deposits of a pigment called bilirubin that comes from the blood. Normally, bilirubin is excreted via the liver into the stool and it gives stool its yellow color. (Food pigments then add the brown color.) When bilirubin is not processed by the liver this way, it yellows the skin and the whites of the eyes, and turns the urine a dark reddish-brown.

### Abdominal Swelling (Ascites)

Swelling of the abdomen can give rise to difficulty breathing, inability to eat a full meal and a sensation of bloating. The fluid retention causing the swelling of the abdomen is caused by the cirrhotic liver "telling" the kidneys not to get rid of salt as they usually do. So the body retains salt, and water as well, so that you do not turn into a rock of salt. A salt-restricted diet is necessary to control water buildup. The doctor may also give you water pills (diuretics) to help you excrete the accumulated fluid.

In more severe cases, a procedure called *paracentesis* is performed: a needle is inserted through the skin of your abdomen to remove the fluid. Sometimes a medical emergency arises when the fluid becomes infected. Any patient with fluid in the abdomen and abdominal pain and/or fever should go to the emergency room immediately.

*High Blood Pressure in the Portal Vein (Portal Hypertension)*
Scarring of the liver slows down the blood that flows through the liver. This causes the blood to back up into the portal vein, the main vein going to the liver, so the blood pressure in the portal vein increases. With increasing obstruction of the flow of blood to the liver, the blood backs up in the spleen (located on the upper left side of the belly). As a result, the spleen becomes congested and increases in size, which is called *splenomegaly*. This condition is associated with a fall in the components of your blood—platelets, white blood cells and hemoglobin. Platelets are needed to help blood clot, white blood cells are needed to fight infection and a loss of red blood cells causes anemia and fatigue.

*Bleeding from Enlarged Vessels (Variceal Bleeding)*
Portal hypertension can lead to another complication—bleeding from the enlarged vessels in the esophagus. When the blood flow to the liver is blocked because of scar tissue, the blood bypasses the liver and finds its way back to the heart via smaller vessels around the esophagus and the stomach. When these small vessels dilate (expand) to the point where they cannot hold the pressure any longer, they will burst and start to bleed. This can be a life-threatening emergency.

If you have hepatitis C and established cirrhosis, the specialist (generally a gastroenterologist) will suggest a check for the presence of enlarged vessels in the esophagus on a regular basis—about every two to three years—via gastroscopy. Gastroscopy is a procedure in which a flexible tube is introduced through the mouth into the esophagus and the stomach. The procedure is generally done under sedation, but it can still be a little bit uncomfortable. However, it is essential that people with cirrhosis have this done to identify their risk of a future variceal bleed. The bigger the vessels, the greater the chance of spontaneous rupture and bleeding. Once large vessels are found, the doctor will prescribe a high-blood-pressure pill called a beta-blocker to lower the blood pressure in the portal vein and reduce the risk of rupture and bleeding. Signs of variceal bleeding include vomiting fresh blood and passing of black "tarry" stools. If you have either of these, it is essential to get to the nearest emergency room immediately.

## Personality Changes and Mental Confusion (Hepatic Encephalopathy)

As the cirrhotic liver deteriorates, its ability to detoxify and filter the blood is decreased. In addition, much of the blood bypasses the liver and travels back to the heart via smaller vessels, so that this blood is no longer being filtered. Toxins normally destroyed by the liver get carried by the blood to the brain.

Family members may notice a change in the person's personality, and the individual may have difficulty sleeping at night, and complain of nightmares and a tendency to sleep during the day. Later still, disorientation, confusion, forgetfulness and an inability to concentrate will develop. If not treated promptly, the person may lapse into a coma. The doctor will prescribe a medication called *lactulose* to relieve this symptom. This sweet yellow medicine is very helpful, but it causes gas and diarrhea. Once a bout of hepatic encephalopathy has occurred, driving a vehicle is prohibited.

Some people who have hepatitis C but no cirrhosis notice a problem with concentration and learning new tasks. The reason for this is at present unknown—it may or may not be caused by their hepatitis C infection—but it is *not* related to the severity of their liver disease.

### *Easy Bruising (Coagulopathy)*
Easy bruising is caused by a combination of low platelets and low clotting factor in the blood. Other signs of these deficiencies include bleeding gums and nosebleeds. Note, however, that elderly people who bruise easily do not necessarily have liver disease.

## Liver Cancer
Primary liver cancer, or *hepatocellular carcinoma*, is one of the most common human malignancies worldwide, although it is less common in North America, affecting 2 to 5 people out of 100,000. Among the most common risk factors for the development of this cancer are viral hepatitis—especially hepatitis B and hepatitis C—and cirrhosis from any cause. In hepatitis C, liver cancer almost exclusively develops in people with liver cirrhosis. It has been estimated that among those with cirrhosis due to hepatitis C, the incidence of liver cancer is between 1 and 5 percent per year. There is some suggestion that interferon therapy—even if eradication of the virus does not occur—may decrease the risk of liver cancer among people with cirrhosis and hepatitis C virus infection, although this remains to be fully proven.

It is now known that, as soon as cirrhosis is established in someone with hepatitis C, there is the risk of developing liver cancer. You don't have to have liver failure—any of the problems just described—before you develop liver cancer. The risk is highest if you are a male over the age of 55, continue to drink alcohol or are infected with hepatitis B as well as hepatitis C.

Owing to the large size of the liver, cancers are often completely without symptoms except in advanced stages. But when liver cancer is advanced, the therapeutic options are limited and often ineffective. Screening for liver cancer using ultrasound is usually done every six months, and any suspicious abnormalities are further investigated with other diagnostic tests.

A blood test called *alpha-fetoprotein (AFP)* can be used as a screening test for liver cancer, but it is not very reliable because people with active hepatitis C without cancer commonly have high levels of AFP in their blood. Nevertheless, your doctor may order this screening test, and/or a regular ultrasound examination of your liver, if you have cirrhosis. However, there is no recommendation at the present time that routine screening for liver cancer should be done on everyone infected with hepatitis C, or even on those with cirrhosis. Treatment with interferon appears to have some protective effect against the development of liver cancer.

It is probable that the detection and treatment of small tumors is associated with a better chance of successful treatment—that is, improved survival—but this has never been proven. If discovered early, liver cancer can be treated surgically, either by removing the tumorous portion of the liver or by liver transplant. There are also non-surgical techniques that can destroy small tumors, such as radiofrequency ablation (in which the tumor is pulverized by high-frequency sound waves) or the injection of strong alcohol.

## Complications of Cryoglobulinemia
Fortunately, symptomatic cryoglobulinemia (see Chapter 1) is quite rare (affecting less than 1 percent of those who have

chronic hepatitis C). The most common complaint is the inter-mittent appearance of small (pinpoint) to large (pea-sized) red blotches, most noticeable on the lower legs. When the blotches fade, the skin is left with a brown stain. These blotches do not hurt and rarely itch.

Cryoglobulinemia can cause kidney problems that result in swelling of the legs. Another symptom is painful tingling of the legs, and sometimes also of the arms. This is due to nerve damage from the cryoglobulins, which have caused inflam-mation of small blood vessels that supply the nerves. It is now recognized that, in people who have cryoglobulinemia, exam-ination of the bone marrow shows lymphoma 25 to 40 percent of the time. Lymphoma is a malignancy of the white blood cells that can be associated with hepatitis C. The symptoms are vague, much like those of uncomplicated hepatitis C. Recent studies indicate that lymphomas associated with hepatitis C respond well to treatment with interferon, and that this treatment may be preferable to standard chemotherapy.

# FIVE

# Treatment and Side Effects

There are two main reasons to try antiviral treatment (medications that fight viruses) for hepatitis C.

- to get rid of symptoms so you can feel better, which is the main goal for those who have symptoms
- to prevent the liver from deteriorating by eradicating the virus

As long as the virus remains present, further damage to the liver is possible. Antiviral therapy is one of the things that can help stop this. It is unlikely that the virus will disappear without antiviral therapy.

Currently, only two forms of therapy have been approved by Canada's Health Protection Bureau and the Federal Drug Administration of the U.S.A. The alpha interferons were the first to be licensed. There are several forms: interferon alpha 2a (Roferon), interferon alpha 2b (Intron A) and interferon alpha-con-1 (Infergen). Later, Rebetron, a combination of interferon alpha 2b and ribavirin, was licensed, and it is now the "standard of care" for adults, though not for children. All interferons need to be given by injection with a tiny needle inserted just under the skin, or with a special "gun" similar to the one used by people with diabetes who require regular injections of insulin. Ribavirin comes in pill form to be taken by mouth.

## Who Should Consider Antiviral Treatment?

Antiviral therapy is generally only recommended when someone with hepatitis C has liver enzyme values (ALT) in the blood that remain elevated for several months in a row. Not everyone who is infected with hepatitis C has abnormal liver blood tests. Although most people with hepatitis C who have normal ALT values test positive for HCV RNA—that is, test positive for the actual virus—some test negative. In children infected with hepatitis C, nearly 50 percent are cleared of the virus without treatment; in adults, only 15 percent to 30 percent lose the virus spontaneously.

No antiviral treatment is necessary if the HCV RNA test is negative.

## The Chances of a Cure

The cure rates—which means the chance of permanently losing detectable virus (HCV RNA) from the blood—are increasing as treatments improve. The best treatment to date, Rebetron, leads to a cure in about 40 percent of those completing a course of treatment. The cure rate with Rebetron therapy depends on several factors, of which genotype is the most important:

- the virus genotype: 1, 2, 3, 4, 5 or 6 (see Chapter 2)
- the amount of virus in the blood (viral load)
- the severity of the underlying liver disease
- the person's weight and height
- whether the person is male or female
- the duration of the infection

A simple blood test that examines the actual virus will identify both the genotype and the viral load. Most laboratories in the U.S.A. conduct these tests, and regional public health laboratories are gearing up to make these tests available to Canadians who are considering antiviral treatments.

Women are more likely to respond to the treatment than men. People who are treated near the time when they first become infected, and who are younger than 40, are more likely to be clear of the virus after therapy. Recently, it has been recognized that markedly overweight people respond poorly to treatment. If the liver is already scarred, treatment is a little more risky and the chance of success is a little lower. However, this does not mean that people with cirrhosis should not be offered antiviral therapy; they should be, as long as there are no contraindications. Knowing all these factors can help to predict the likelihood of a response to Rebetron therapy—but if none or only some of these "good" factors are present, the idea of treatment certainly should not be abandoned. The decision as to whether or not to go for treatment will be easier if you know these factors, the presence or absence of relative contraindications to treatment and, finally, whether the timing is convenient.

## When Is Antiviral Treatment Considered Unsafe?

There is no medication, even ASA, that does not have side effects. Side effects can often be predicted based on how the drug is eliminated from the body.

- Ribavirin (one of the two drugs in Rebetron) is removed from the body via the kidneys, in the urine. Therefore, this medication cannot be given to anyone who has poor kidney function, because the drug will build up to toxic levels in the body.

- Ribavirin can cause the red blood cells to die before the end of their usual 120-day lifespan. Death of a lot of red blood cells all at once results in the sudden onset of anemia. If you are quite healthy apart from hepatitis C, this sudden anemia is not a major problem. But for people who already have problems with anemia that cannot be treated—for example, thalassemia—a further fall in blood count can be dangerous.

- Because red blood cells carry oxygen, ribavirin should not be given to anyone whose body would not tolerate a sudden fall in oxygen supply—for example, someone who has heart problems, or problems with the blood vessels to the brain.

- Interferon (IFN) therapy is not advised for those who have or have had severe mental illness that has caused them to hallucinate or to contemplate suicide, even if these problems were a long time in the past. As well, IFN can affect the brain in people who have epilepsy, so they should be on medication to control their seizures prior to starting IFN therapy.

- It is never a good idea to take any medication during pregnancy unless it is medically necessary. When taken *by either males or females*, ribavirin is associated with an increase in the death rate of babies conceived during the treatment or within six months of stopping treatment. So unless both partners can be confident that conception will not occur, Rebetron therapy—and probably even IFN alone—should not be used.

- In persons who have already developed scarring of the liver to the point of having cirrhosis, the levels of white cells and/or platelets in the blood are often reduced. As IFN tends to reduce the ability of the body to make both white blood cells and platelets, IFN therapy should not be used if the levels are too low. Whereas a sudden fall in the platelet count is rarely serious, a sudden fall in the white blood cell count could put you at risk of a serious, even fatal, bacterial infection throughout the blood (septicemia).

It is very important that, before prescribing hepatitis C treatment with any medication, the doctor knows all the current and past medical problems of the patient. Further consultation with other physicians may be necessary at this point.

## When Is Antiviral Treatment Considered Unwise?

Interferons are natural substances that the body produces to fight viral infections, and the side effects of IFN treatment are similar to those of the flu—fever, muscle aches, headaches, loss of appetite and depression. Most of these side effects fade after the first few injections. But if you are depressed before starting treatment, it is wise to discuss the possibility of taking antidepressant medication prior to the IFN therapy.

Certain conditions can be activated or made worse by treatment with IFN. These conditions are

- thyroid disease
- diabetes
- psoriasis
- lichen planus of the skin
- any autoimmune disease—for example, systemic lupus erythematosus, rheumatoid arthritis, autoimmune hepatitis, ulcerative colitis or Crohn's disease

*Thyroid disease* can be controlled with medication, so thyroid levels should be checked intermittently during therapy with IFN.

---

**Antiviral medications for hepatitis C**

| | |
|---|---|
| Rebetron: | interferon alpha 2b plus ribavirin |
| Roferon: | interferon alpha 2a |
| Intron A: | interferon alpha 2b |
| Infergen: | interferon alpha-con-1 |

---

*Diabetes* may become difficult to control during IFN therapy, because the drug affects the level of blood sugar.

*Psoriasis* is a common and troublesome skin condition (not caused by hepatitis C). If it is present before the treatment, it can spread to all parts of the body after the start of IFN therapy. If this happens, the treatment must be stopped.

*Lichen planus* is a skin condition associated with hepatitis C that frequently gets worse during therapy with IFN. This may cause severe discomfort, particularly if there are skin lesions in the mouth or vagina.

If in addition to your hepatitis C you have an *autoimmune disease*, consult the doctor taking care of this condition prior to starting any antiviral treatment. If, during the course of the next year, treatment with prednisone or other immunosuppressive therapy is likely—for example, for recurrent bouts of asthma—it is probably not worthwhile considering treatment for hepatitis C. This is because medicines like steroids cause the hepatitis C virus to multiply so much that the antiviral therapy just cannot do its job.

## How to Decide

Once you and your doctor have discussed whether some form of antiviral treatment is safe for you, it's time for the next phase in the decision-making process.

### Other Factors to Consider

Many people consider the side effects of therapy to be greater than any perceived benefit. But as the side effects cannot be predicted in any particular person, it may be a good idea to at least try therapy, and discontinue or continue it depending on how well you tolerate it.

There are times when the liver damage is so mild that it's safe to hold off therapy until a better treatment comes on the market. A liver biopsy can be performed to assess the severity of disease.

### Weighing the Pros and Cons

Each individual needs to decide when and if the therapies currently available for hepatitis are worthwhile. Weigh the benefits against the costs to get an indication of how likely it is that the therapy will be a positive experience for you.

Remember that the costs of therapy are not simply any bills you pay at the pharmacy. They include the blood tests needed to monitor treatment, and the time a nurse or physician spends overseeing the treatment. Fortunately, many of these costs are covered under various health insurance plans. But a number of indirect personal costs also need to be considered.

- Is this a time in my life when I can commit to undergoing repeated blood tests and visits to the doctor's office for up to a year?
- How is this therapy going to affect my work performance and productivity, or my relationships with my spouse, family and friends?
- Do I really need this now? Treatment with the currently available therapies cannot be taken lightly, especially if I have additional illnesses.
- I'm young now. However, even if my infection with hepatitis C is mild at the time of my first liver biopsy, it may eventually have an impact on my health.

Perhaps you can afford to wait for better treatments in the future. It will be very important to keep in regular contact with your doctor in the meantime, as our understanding of hepatitis C is growing all the time.

If you decide not to go for therapy for now, a repeat liver biopsy in about three years is recommended, to make sure the hepatitis is not progressing. If it is found to be progressing, you can then start the best treatment available at that time.

## The Significance of the Genotype

There are several genotypes of the hepatitis C virus, and most people are infected with only one. The particular genotype of your hepatitis C virus predicts only the likelihood of cure with therapy, not the severity of the disease. The majority (more than 60 percent) of North Americans with hepatitis C are infected with genotype 1a or 1b, and unfortunately these are the most resistant to current therapies. Genotypes 2 and 3 are the forms that respond best to treatment.

## The Significance of the Viral Load

The amount of virus present in your blood may be used to decide how long antiviral treatment should be given—e.g., for six or twelve months. The amount of virus circulating in any one person tends to remain stable over long periods of time unless:

- prednisone and/or other immunosuppressive therapy (anticancer or antirejection medications) are used
- any kind of alcohol (beer, wine or hard liquor) is drunk on a regular basis, even if the drinking is not excessive

Levels of greater than 2 to 3.5 million copies of virus/milliliter of blood are considered high. (Starting in 2001, the virus load is being measured in iu/liter, but this cannot be translated to the old system. However, most references you come across will still be to copies of virus per milliliter.) Successful cure following treatment is much more likely if the viral load is low before treatment, rather than high.

**What Are My Chances of Being Cured?**
It is important to realize that, when new drugs for any disease are being evaluated, there are always very strict rules about who is allowed to enter these studies. You have to be cautious about interpreting the results—particularly if, for whatever reason, you would not have been eligible for the studies. Although the published results of the studies are true for those who were in the studies, we don't know if the same treatment will be equally effective in others with hepatitis C. Bear this in mind, and also recognize that these studies were performed mostly on middle-aged white men with quite mild liver disease, persistently abnormal liver enzyme (ALT) levels in their blood, and no co-infection with HIV or hepatitis B.

The success rates—that is, the rates of people being cured—depend greatly upon the genotype of the virus.

- Success rates for genotype 1 range from 25 to 30 percent.
- Success rates for genotypes 2 and 3 range from 60 to 70 percent.
- For other genotypes, the cure rates are somewhere between those for genotype 1 and genotypes 2 and 3.

## What Happens If I Opt for Treatment?
Once you have decided that antiviral treatment is appropriate, several tubes of your blood will be taken to make sure that it is safe for you to start. These tests are for:

- level of white blood cells
- level of platelets

- level of red blood cells (hemoglobin)
- level of blood sugar
- function of the kidneys
- function of the thyroid
- liver enzyme values
- HIV
- pregnancy (for premenopausal females)

### When Should I Start Treatment?

Because the side effects are most frequent within the first two weeks of starting therapy, it is important to choose a time when it is possible for you to take life a little easy. Students are advised not to start treatment just before examinations, for example, and it is not sensible to start treatment at the same time as beginning a new job.

### Monitoring Treatment

Regular blood tests will be required every week for at least the first month, and perhaps longer, and then at least every month for the duration of treatment (six to twelve months depending on the genotype). It is helpful to avoid frequent trips away from your home town during treatment.

The results of these blood tests will be used as a guide to decide whether the dose of the interferon and/or the ribavirin needs to be reduced or perhaps even stopped—for example, when the side effects on the white blood cells and/or platelets and/or hemoglobin are too severe. Of course, severe symptoms alone may indicate the need to change doses, but blood tests are also essential. It is vital that the nurse or doctor monitoring your therapy be able to contact you by telephone at any time, to discuss the results of blood tests or leave you instructions. Therefore you must have an answering machine, cellphone (switched on!), pager or answering service.

**Habits That Will Reduce Your Chance of a Cure**

Because the regular drinking of alcohol (beer, wine, liquor, etc.) causes an increase in the amount of virus circulating in your blood, it makes no sense to undergo treatment unless you are willing to abstain from all alcohol consumption.

Continued use of injected or "snorted" street drugs will permit re-infection with hepatitis C, so there is no point going for therapy until this habit has been stopped.

# Treatment of Hepatitis C in Children

There have now been a number of studies on the effects of contracting hepatitis C in childhood (generally through a transfusion of blood or blood products when the child was very young). In those who did not manage to eliminate the virus on their own, the severity of liver disease tended to be mild in most but not all cases. Figures indicate that after twenty years of infection, 1 to 8 percent will have cirrhosis of the liver, and about 20 percent will have some mild scarring of the liver.

There are encouraging data to suggest that hepatitis C in children may run a milder course than infection acquired in adulthood. In children exposed to the virus through blood transfusion, the infection appeared to resolve on its own more often (45 to 50 percent of cases) than in adults (15 to 30 percent). As well, examination of liver tissue taken by biopsy shows very little fibrosis, although exceptions do occur.

Although there is reason for cautious optimism about the outcome of hepatitis C virus infection in children, this must be tempered by the fact that the published studies are few, and followup is limited to ten to twenty years; it is known that the infection may persist for life and progress over decades.

Children with hepatitis C tolerate antiviral treatment much better than do adults. There was some concern that their growth might be interrupted, particularly if treatment was given during a growth spurt, but it seems that this concern is probably unfounded. At present, however, the standard treatment recommended for adults cannot be used for children, because Rebetron is not licensed for use in children in Canada or the U.S.A.

## Co-infection with Another Virus

### Hepatitis C and HIV

In Chapter 4 it was pointed out that liver disease progresses more rapidly in people with hepatitis C if they are co-infected with HIV. Now that the treatment for HIV has so markedly improved, it is becoming even more urgent that good therapies for hepatitis C be found for those infected with both viruses. Unfortunately there have been few trials reporting on the benefit of alpha interferon alone. But some data show that in a person whose HIV infection is well controlled, the response to this therapy can be as good as it is in someone who has hepatitis C alone. In addition, once treatment for the hepatitis C is stopped, the relapse rate does not seem to be any greater.

There is little known currently of the benefits or safety of Rebetron therapy in those with hepatitis C as well as HIV, although plenty of trials are ongoing. There is justified concern that there may be some risks to using Rebetron in those being treated for HIV at the same time. Anyone undergoing treatment for both viruses has to be watched very, very carefully during antiviral therapy.

### Hepatitis C and Hepatitis B

Fortunately it is most unusual for both hepatitis C and B to be active at the same time. It is important for your doctor to

## Common side effects of antiviral treatment

- flu-like symptoms (headaches, fever, chills and fatigue)
- muscle and joint aches
- decreased appetite and nausea (metallic taste)
- difficulty sleeping (insomnia)
- dry, itchy skin
- hair loss
- irritability
- depression
- shortness of breath *(dyspnea)*
- diarrhea
- mouth ulcers

determine from blood tests which virus is active and therefore which one needs to be treated. Although it may involve the use of interferon, the treatment for hepatitis B is different from the treatment for hepatitis C. Standard guidelines for treating hepatitis B are not yet established, as many new treatments are currently being assessed in clinical trials.

## Side Effects

Antiviral treatment can affect people both physically and psychologically. These are the most common side effects.

At the very start of the treatment, flu-like symptoms (headache, fever, chills and fatigue), muscle and joint aches, decreased appetite, nausea and insomnia affect the majority of people, but they usually diminish with time. Later side effects, which fortunately occur less frequently, are dry itchy skin, hair loss and psychological effects, particularly irritability and depression. The severity and type of side effects differ for each individual and these side effects disappear soon after the medication is discontinued. Side effects of interferon treatment fade very rapidly once the therapy stops, usually beginning within 36 hours, and all are gone within a week.

Because ribavirin lasts within the body for a lot longer than interferon, its side effects—mostly fatigue and potential damage to an unborn baby—can persist for weeks.

It is essential to inform your doctor or nurse of any side effects you are experiencing, so that they can give you additional advice on coping with your symptoms more effectively. Adjustment of your dose of therapy may be required. If the side effects are severe and become intolerable, you can always stop the treatment. Remember, treatment is supposed to help, not harm you!

### Flu-like Symptoms

The best way to cope with these symptoms, which are experienced as early as the first day of treatment and generally lessen thereafter, is to eat a well-balanced diet, drink plenty of water, exercise regularly and try hard to be as productive as possible. If the symptoms become severe and you cannot tolerate the side effects, acetaminophen can be taken every four to six hours or prior to injecting the interferon, to minimize the severity of the symptoms.

How you deal with the flu-like symptoms right at the beginning of the treatment has some impact on your ability to tolerate the treatment later. If you choose to deal with these symptoms by going to bed, your productivity will fall off and undone tasks will start to accumulate. This in turn causes a buildup of stress, and depression may result from your lack of productivity. If you ignore this response, you may progress to a feeling of uselessness, and even to destructive behavior. So it is best to cope with these flu-like symptoms right from the beginning. If they cause some restrictions in your everyday activities, you may want to consider taking the antiviral medication at bedtime, so that most of the effects occur while you are asleep.

## Muscle and Joint Aches

Exercise is a key factor in improving muscle and joint aches and controlling stress. It can also lessen the severity and frequency of headaches. However, listen to your body for signals as to how much activity it can tolerate. If you set your goals too high, and they are unrealistic, your efforts can be counterproductive. It may help to do your exercises with small breaks in between, instead of trying to do everything at once. For example, instead of going for an hour's walk all at once, consider taking fifteen-minute walks with five-minute intervals of rest, sitting on a bench.

Engaging in recreational activity (such as going for a walk with a friend or a dog) also helps to relieve tension and bring on a feeling of relaxation. Exercise always facilitates feelings of self-worth and well-being. Therefore it is very important to keep up as many daily activities as possible, to try to prevent irritability and depression.

Massage therapy can help you relax your mind as well as reduce your muscle aches. You may also want to consider the benefits of a low-impact aerobic class, or yoga or tai chi. Consult your local fitness center for other options.

## Decreased Appetite and Nausea

You may experience a metallic taste in your mouth right after your interferon injection, which in turn may alter your sense of taste and decrease your appetite. Nausea can also occur because of the metallic taste, especially if you are taking Rebetron. Therefore, it is common for people to report a weight loss while on antiviral treatment. Feeling full most of the time, or feeling bloated after eating only a small portion of a meal, is another complaint. It is important that you eat regularly even though you may not be hungry, because your body needs energy to cope with your flu-like symptoms and to carry out routine activities at work and at home. If you do feel nauseated, consider having four or five small meals per day instead of the usual three. You may find that your food preferences change. Fresh fruit, fish, chicken and bland foods may be more appealing than red meat or cheese products. Some people find that cold food is easier to consume. Prepare your food according to what appeals to your appetite, in order to keep up a healthy diet.

### Insomnia

You may have difficulty sleeping as soon as you start antiviral treatment. One of the common reasons for insomnia is simply the anticipation of potential side effects! Listening to music or reading a book may help you relax. Other techniques, like having a massage or taking a warm bath at bedtime, can help relax your muscles and your mind, and hence promote better sleep.

### Dry, Itchy Skin

Not only can increased fluid intake (two to three quarts [liters] per day) help you to cope with flu-like symptoms at the beginning of your treatment, it can also help you avoid the dry skin that can occur toward the end of the treatment. It is better to prevent this side effect by drinking water as soon as the treatment is started than to wait for the symptom to show up. It is best to drink most of the fluid during the day, and minimize your fluid intake after dinner, to prevent interruption of your sleep. If you do experience dry, itchy skin, applying a moisturizer to your body often helps. It is important that you inform your doctor or nurse as well, so that they can check for other skin problems associated with antiviral treatment. There can on very rare occasions be an unpleasant, serious skin reaction at the injection site.

**Tips on handling side effects**
- Eat a well-balanced diet.
- Drink plenty of fluids.
- Exercise regularly.
- Be productive.

## Hair Loss

Hair loss is quite a common side effect of interferon, and this can affect your self-image. The loss is only temporary and never total, and the hair will return to normal after treatment is discontinued. If this symptom is going to develop, it usually starts about two months into treatment; it lasts for three to four months after that. However, the hair may not regrow until treatment is stopped. It is highly unlikely that you will go bald and need a wig, as sometimes happens with chemotherapy. While you are on the treatment and experiencing hair loss, you may want to consider a shorter haircut so that the loss is less noticeable. Keep in mind that a perm or coloring can weaken your hair and cause more hair loss, so these are not recommended during the treatment.

## Irritability

Irritability is a psychological side effect experienced, to varying degrees, by many people during antiviral therapy. You should seek help when you cannot control your temper. Sometimes it is other household members who are most aware of such changes in personality, and they may need to come along with you to your followup visits to discuss the changes. Unfortunately there is no treatment for irritability on its own. Just remember that the side effects are only temporary!

## Depression

Depression is the symptom that most commonly causes people to stop therapy. The best way to prevent depression is by dealing with the flu-like symptoms effectively in the beginning of the treatment. However, not everyone can prevent the depression. It is important to know that there are very good medications to combat depression. If you know that you tend to have a low mood on occasion, it may be advisable to take a prescription antidepressant medication throughout the time you are on antiviral treatment. There is no danger in doing this, and it may make it much easier for you to complete therapy.

## Shortness of Breath (Dyspnea)

Ribavirin can cause a fall in your red blood cell count (hemoglobin). As your red blood cells carry oxygen, a decrease in your hemoglobin means that there is less oxygen available for your body. This may cause you to feel short of breath, or even faint. If shortness of breath affects your daily activities, it is important to inform your doctor or nurse of the way you feel; they will likely adjust your dose of ribavirin. If you feel faint, you may find yourself slowing down. Try to sit up slowly before standing up from a lying position, otherwise you may feel dizzy and faint. Shortness of breath may begin anytime during treatment, and it may take you weeks to adjust to it. The problem is especially noticeable with exertion. Your doctor or nurse will let you know when it is appropriate to reduce the number of ribavirin pills, based on the results of your blood tests. Never be afraid to tell them about your symptoms.

## Diarrhea

The onset of loose stools is often noticed at the beginning of the interferon treatment, together with the flu-like symptoms, and usually lasts for one or two months. Rarely, diarrhea continues throughout the course of treatment. When diarrhea is a problem it is particularly important to increase your daily fluid intake to at least three quarts (liters) per day, to avoid dehydration. If you do get diarrhea, you may find it helpful to avoid milk and milk products until the diarrhea is resolved. There is generally no need to change your diet in other ways, although it would be unwise to eat excessive amounts of fruit.

## Mouth Ulcers

Mouth ulcers are a relatively rare side effect with interferon alone, but they are more likely when ribavirin is added to the regimen. They may develop at any time during treatment. If they do appear, you may find some foods hard to eat, especially fresh fruit, raw vegetables, tough meat and hot or sour food. You may want to consider eating soft fruits (such as bananas), steamed vegetables and ground meat. Milk or milk-shakes are recommended as they are high in calories and protein, but do not use these as replacements for all your meals. It is important to wash your mouth after meals, and to drink plenty of fluid during the day to keep your mouth moist and comfortable. As with any other side effects, consult your physician or nurse immediately, particularly so that your weight can be monitored. Your doctor may prescribe high-calorie/high-protein liquid or powdered dietary supplements, if required.

Carlos, who is 35 years old and works as a computer technician, was diagnosed with hepatitis C two years ago. Although he was feeling well, his blood tests showed persistently elevated liver transaminase values, so treatment was recommended.

Carlos had read on the Internet that interferon treatment can have severe side effects. At first he did not want to consider treatment, mainly because his job requires concentration and a high energy level every day. He would have preferred to be off work during the period of treatment, but he could not afford that because he was supporting a wife and two young children.

At the many visits when his prognosis was discussed, Carlos learned that everyone's body is different and that not everyone who receives treatment will suffer all the side effects described on the Internet. With the reassurance that he would be closely monitored, Carlos decided to go for treatment, starting during his summer vacation. He experienced some headaches, chills and fever after his interferon injections during the first week, but few problems after that, except for thinning of his hair.

Carlos was advised to take regular or extra-strength acetaminophen after the injection, and on the next morning, to help relieve his flu-like symptoms. He was also advised to increase his fluid intake to three quarts (liters) per day. He was surprised that by the time he restarted work he could deal well with the treatment. This was likely because he has always been physically active, and exercise lifts his spirits. He tolerated the treatment well, and was happy that he had finally agreed to it. He was even happier when he learned that he had responded well, and that hepatitis C was no longer detectable in his blood.

# What If I Don't Respond to Antiviral Therapy?

There comes a time when it is possible to predict whether the treatment is working or not. Measurement of the ALT level is not very reliable, so the blood must be checked to see whether or not the hepatitis C virus RNA can still be detected. It is still unclear exactly when this test should be performed, but if the HCV RNA test is still positive 24 weeks into treatment, then you are definitely a *non-responder*. (A non-responder is someone who continues to have detectable HCV RNA despite therapy with either IFN alone or IFN with ribavirin.)

You may be quite disappointed at being a non-responder, but you must realize that this is *not* a death sentence—the progression to severe disease in those who remain infected with hepatitis C is generally very, very slow, and in any case it does not happen in everyone.

When we say that someone has "responded" because the virus is "undetectable" in the blood, all we are saying is that the viral load is so low that current testing cannot detect it. The more sensitive our testing becomes, the more accurate our results will be. Currently the lower limit of detectability is about 100 copies of the virus in a milliliter of blood, which is very low, but tests are being developed that will pick up an even smaller amount of the virus. This means that, in the future, it may be possible to determine even earlier if you are a non-responder, by measuring how much the viral load falls after you start therapy.

### Can a Cure Be Predicted during Treatment?

Unfortunately, the answer to this question at present is no. Even though the HCV RNA may become undetectable during treatment, a relapse can occur when the treatment is stopped. Right now, relapse or cure cannot be forecast; we can only determine whether someone is a responder or a non-responder. If the HCV RNA test shows that the virus is undetectable six months after you complete the course of therapy, there is a 95 percent chance that you are cured; that is, you are a *sustained responder*.

Oscar went for an insurance physical when he was 33 years old. Although he felt fine, he was asked to go and see his family physician, because his blood tests indicated some abnormality with his liver. His liver tests remained elevated even after he took his physician's advice and gave up his usual three to four beers a night. In the course of further investigation, his hepatitis C test came back positive, and he was referred to a specialist who advised a liver biopsy to assess the degree of liver damage. The biopsy showed severe inflammation and scarring, but no cirrhosis.

As Oscar had no contraindications to treatment, he was started on Rebetron. His viral load was high and he was geno-type 1a so it was decided that he would require treatment for 48 weeks. Initially his blood was checked weekly, and all the test results remained within a safe range, so the full dose of treatment was continued and blood tests were required only monthly. However, even though Oscar's liver enzymes returned to normal, a recheck of his HCV RNA three months into treatment showed that it remained detectable.

Oscar decided to continue treatment for another three months, hoping that he would be one of the few (8 percent) who fail to clear the virus after three months of Rebetron but manage to clear the virus after six months. But his HCV RNA test was still positive after six months of Rebetron, so he was advised to stop therapy at that point.

Because Oscar had not suffered many side effects during treatment, he was anxious to continue with therapy. His doctor explained that it was unlikely continued treatment would clear the virus, although some data indicated that, even in a non-responder like Oscar, the liver inflammation might improve. It was explained to him, however, that the data were not sufficiently convincing to suggest that continued therapy was the best thing for him.

Oscar's doctor advised him to continue avoiding alcohol, and encouraged him to quit smoking and to start leading a healthier lifestyle, including a balanced diet and regular exercise. His doctor also reminded him that, although he had evidence of progressive disease, the progression is very slow in hepatitis C. The doctor advised regular checkups, and emphasized that there would be more effective medications available for hepatitis C in the not-too-distant future, so Oscar should keep in touch with his physician.

## What about Relapses?

If you lose detectable virus in your blood during treatment for your hepatitis C, but when treatment is stopped the virus reappears, you have had a *relapse*.

There are two equally effective options for re-treating people who have relapsed following *interferon treatment given on its own*, which was the standard treatment until 1998–1999. These options are

- to treat again, with combination therapy—that is, Rebetron, if there is no contraindication; chance of cure, 49 percent
- otherwise, to treat again with IFN alpha-con-1 (Infergen), using a large dose three times a week; chance of cure, 59 percent

Whereas the relapse rate after initial treatment with interferon alone is close to 50 percent, the relapse rate following Rebetron is only about 25 percent. Relapse is generally associated with recurrence of abnormal liver enzyme values, and may or may not be associated with symptoms. If it is going to occur, relapse generally takes place within three months of stopping treatment, but it can be much later. There is currently no recommendation for treatment of relapse following Rebetron therapy.

Susan had known since 1990 that her blood tests for liver enzymes were elevated, but no diagnosis had been made until 1991, when testing for hepatitis C became available. At that time she read in the paper that if someone had had a blood transfusion prior to 1991, this could cause infection with hepatitis C. This worried her, as she had needed a transfusion because of a miscarriage in 1980. She asked her family doctor for the hepatitis C test, and she tested positive.

Susan had never been a drinker and she was otherwise quite well, apart from some fatigue which she put down to having four teenagers at home. However, she had noticed a purplish-red patch on her wrist. She was referred to a specialist who advised that she undergo a liver biopsy. The biopsy showed mild inflammation and almost no scarring, and Susan was told that treatment was not vital at that time. But Susan was very anxious to get rid of the hepatitis C because she felt she was putting her family at risk, even though her doctor explained that the chance of her passing the infection on to her husband and children was very slim. (They had all been tested, and were negative for hepatitis C.)

Treatment was started with interferon alone in 1992, when there were no other treatments available. Susan tolerated the treatment well and was delighted that her liver tests returned to normal almost immediately after. At the end of six months the treatment was stopped. (No testing for HCV RNA was available at that time.) Shortly after she finished her treatment, blood tests showed a flare-up of her liver enzymes, although she had not noticed any new symptom development. Naturally she was very disappointed. Again she was reassured that, because she had only mild hepatitis, it was unlikely anything too serious would happen to her in the near future.

In 1997, after reading on a website that twelve months of IFN treatment was more likely to result in a cure, Susan asked to be treated again. This time she was given double her original dose of IFN and treated for a full year. Once again her liver blood tests returned to normal soon after she started therapy. Her HCV RNA was tested at the end of three months of treatment. It was undetectable, and has remained so ever since she completed her year of treatment. Susan's healthcare team has explained to her that she has a 95 percent chance of remaining cured for the rest of her life, unless she becomes re-exposed to the virus in some way.

### What Does It Mean to Be a "Sustained Responder"?

If, when your blood is checked six months after the completion of treatment, HCV RNA remains undetectable in your blood, there is a 95 percent chance that the virus has gone for good and that there will be no further deterioration of the liver; in fact, there is likely to be a gradual improvement, although cirrhosis itself is unlikely to disappear.

Because you cannot acquire long-lasting immunity to hepatitis C, it is entirely possible for you to become infected again. Returning to a risky lifestyle that might expose you to the virus again, such as intravenous drug use, cocaine "snorting," tattoos or body piercing, is obviously unwise.

## Will All the Symptoms Go Away?

Symptoms that are specific to the hepatitis C infection—for example, skin rash, kidney problems or symptoms of cryoglobulinemia caused by the hepatitis C virus—will disappear when you are free of the hepatitis C virus.

The effect on the other, more non-specific symptoms that appear in some but not all people with hepatitis C is unpredictable. Vitality is restored in some people, but not in all. If you get rid of your hepatitis C virus you will probably feel much better, but it is not wise to expect every symptom to disappear completely.

## Long-term Effects of Antiviral Therapy

In the few patients who have agreed to undergo several repeat liver biopsies after clearing their virus, both the inflammation and the scar tissue in the liver have been reduced. However, it is unlikely that the liver of someone who has had full-blown cirrhosis prior to treatment will return to normal. In those who have cirrhosis and do respond to treatment, complications—for example, fluid in the abdomen—are less likely to occur, and it is possible that the risk of developing liver cancer is reduced.

Indeed, there may be an improvement in the degree of liver inflammation, perhaps even in the degree of liver scarring, in those who are non-responders, despite the fact that the virus is still present.

# SIX

# *Liver Transplantation*

Although hepatitis C has probably been present in humans for a long time, the introduction of remedies given via needle allowed the spread of infected blood from one person to another when unsterile equipment was used. Then, during the 1960s, the use of intravenous illicit drugs became popular. Since users often shared needles, infection spread, and more hepatitis C was introduced into the supply of donor blood. As the contents of one unit of donor blood are distributed to several people, infection with hepatitis C escalated, although we didn't realize it at the time.

Fortunately, only a minority of those infected with hepatitis C develop liver disease so severe that a liver transplant is required. Even so, the number is large enough to far exceed the current supply of donated livers. In the U.S., where hepatitis C is more prevalent (affecting almost 1 percent of the population, compared with 0.8 percent in Canada), hepatitis C is the most common reason for a liver transplant. Not infrequently, the severe liver damage has been promoted by excessive alcohol intake while the person was still unaware of the infection.

## Will I Need a Liver Transplant?

There are two main indications for a liver transplant. The most common is the onset of liver failure; signs include accumulation of fluid in the abdomen, jaundiced eyes, mental confusion, and internal hemorrhage (bleeding) due to rupture of varicose veins in the esophagus.

In addition, anyone with cirrhosis of the liver, due to any cause, is at increased risk of liver cancer. If a cancer is detected when the tumor is small, and there are no more than three tumors present, this too may be reason for a liver transplant.

Not everyone is a suitable candidate for this major surgery. The rest of the body has to be in good enough shape to pull through the surgery. People who continue to smoke are putting themselves at risk of being rejected, because lung and/or heart problems can disqualify someone from receiving a transplant.

Someone being considered for a transplant has to go through a rigorous screening program at a liver transplant center. At the center, the person's case history is presented to a team of physicians, surgeons, nurses and social workers who are all closely involved in the final decision as to whether or not to recommend a liver transplant.

Until recently, the donated liver had to come from someone who had recently died but whose liver was healthy. Now, in some but not all centers, live donor programs have been developed (see below).

## What Is a Liver Transplant?

Liver transplantation is a procedure performed on people who have liver failure and no other treatment options. It is a major operation. The failing liver is removed and replaced with a healthy organ. Most commonly this healthy organ is obtained from a brain-dead individual, in whom the heart and internal organs are still functional but there is no higher brain function and no chance of recovery. Because such unfortunate persons are relatively uncommon, and because not all families of potential organ donors allow the organs to be harvested, the wait for a liver transplant ranges between several months and three years. Organs are allocated based on matching for blood type and size, and are prioritized based on the severity of the potential recipients' medical condition and their length of time on the waiting list.

The liver is unlike other vital organs in that, if a small piece of adult liver is transplanted into someone, it can grow to be a fully functioning organ. Increasingly, transplants are being performed using portions of the livers of living donors. In Canada the law requires such a donor to be a close relative of the person receiving the transplant, such as a parent, brother or sister, or child. This rule is not so strict in the U.S.

A portion of the donor's liver is surgically removed and placed in the recipient to replace the failing organ. Over several weeks, both portions of the healthy liver will grow, so that both the donor and the recipient end up with a normal-sized liver. Potential living donors must be carefully evaluated to minimize the risk of the procedure. The procedure involves a small risk of post-operative complications and even death. (The mortality rate among donors is .025 percent, or 1 in 4,000.)

Upon referral to a liver transplant program, potential recipients also undergo an extensive evaluation to determine that there are no other treatment options available, that they have no anatomical abnormalities that would make transplantation impossible, and that they have no other serious medical conditions that would reduce their chances of surviving the transplant surgery and followup period. The evaluation includes tests to ensure that the heart, lungs and kidneys are functioning well. They must also agree to be followed closely after the transplant, to ensure that the new liver is functioning well and that complications are minimized.

After people are accepted for liver transplantation, their names are placed on a waiting list until their turn comes up and an appropriate organ becomes available. Those on the waiting list are followed closely, and treated aggressively when appropriate, to ensure that they remain in good shape to undergo their transplant. Once an organ becomes available, they are notified to come to the hospital immediately for surgery.

Liver transplantation is performed by specially trained surgeons. The operation takes about six to eight hours. Following the surgery, recipients are transferred to the intensive care unit, where they are cared for by a specialized medical team. After they are sufficiently stable, they are transferred to a ward, and they are usually discharged from hospital within two weeks of the transplant. They are treated with powerful medications to prevent organ rejection but, over time, the frequency and dosage of medications can be reduced.

The goal of liver transplantation is to return the person to a state of good health and to allow a resumption of all normal activities. The overall success rate of the procedure is high: over 90 percent at one year after transplantation, and over 85 percent at five years.

It is hoped that, in the future, the genetic makeup of animals can be altered in such a way that their organs can be accepted by humans, so that there will be no shortage of donor organs. (The pig is the likely candidate.) *Xenotransplantation* is the word used to describe this technique. Xenotransplantation, and other genetic methods whereby new liver cells can be transplanted successfully into humans, are areas of intense medical research.

# Does Hepatitis C Return in the Newly Transplanted Liver?

Unfortunately, the answer is yes. Recurrence of the infection is almost universal, but usually the liver functions well despite the renewed infection, and the five-year survival rate following a liver transplant for chronic hepatitis C is just as good as it is for those who receive a liver transplant for other reasons. In approximately 10 percent of recipients with hepatitis C, the recurrent infection will affect liver function, and special antiviral treatment may be recommended.

We urgently need to find an effective cure that prevents liver failure. Until then, newly transplanted livers will continue to become re-infected. The usual antiviral therapies used to treat hepatitis are poorly tolerated by people who have had transplants, because the anti-rejection (immunosuppressive) therapy necessitated by the transplant causes the virus to multiply actively, thus making it much more difficult to treat. But just as one may have hepatitis C for a long time without knowing it, so the transplanted liver can continue to function normally for many years, despite being re-infected, thus allowing the person to have extra years of life. It would appear that at ten years after transplant the re-infected liver will show some signs of deterioration. Our data at present do not go beyond this time. Hence hepatitis C itself is not a contraindication to receiving a liver transplant.

# SEVEN

## What Can I Do to Help Myself?

epatitis C is still a relatively newly recognized virus infection. The general public lacks knowledge about it, and often incorrectly compares it to other new diseases such as HIV. As a result, there are many myths and misconceptions about hepatitis C. No matter how others see the disease, it is vital for you to know how to take care of yourself so that your life can continue normally. You can keep your health as good as possible, while minimizing the chance of the disease getting worse. Here are some suggestions to help you help yourself.

## Healthy Eating

One common question asked by people with hepatitis C is, "Are there certain kinds of food that I should or should not eat?" There is no magic food that can cure hepatitis C. Although some dietary restrictions are thought necessary, just as they are for people with heart disease and diabetes, there is no need to restrict any specific type of food in your diet,

## How can I best help myself?

- healthy eating—a well-balanced, low-fat, high-fiber diet
- abstinence from alcohol
- regular exercise
- not smoking
- positive mental outlook
- your work
- networking
- caution in taking prescribed and over-the-counter medications
- dietary supplements
- protection against hepatitis A and B
- seeing a liver specialist

unless you have cirrhosis. It is true, however, that how you feel depends in part on what you eat. For example, fatty foods stay in your stomach a long time and may give you a sensation of bloating, but they will not actually damage your liver.

To get the nutrition your body needs, eat a well-balanced, low-fat, high-fiber diet. Your diet should include a balance of meats and/or alternatives (such as fish, eggs, beans), bread and grains, milk products and fruits and vegetables. Changing your way of cooking will help to reduce the amount of fat in your diet. For example, use steaming rather than frying.

As mentioned earlier, when you are nauseated or have a poor appetite it may help to take small, frequent meals instead of three full meals a day, but it is important to meet your body's nutritional needs. If you are overweight, you should engage in a regular exercise program in addition to following a well-balanced diet plan. Too much fat in your body may lead to fatty deposits in your liver (*fatty liver*). Fatty liver causes further inflammation of the liver that can worsen your liver disease. If you have other medical problems, such as diabetes, high blood pressure or high cholesterol, it is best for you to discuss your diet program with your dietitian, doctor or nurse.

People who have developed cirrhosis need to pay particular attention to diet only when symptoms of complications arise. If fluid starts to collect in your abdomen, you must follow a salt-restricted diet. The less salt (sodium) you take in your diet, the better you will be able to control the amount of fluid in your abdomen. Make sure to read all food labels when you are shopping for groceries. Condiments such as ketchup, mustard and soya sauce usually have a high sodium content, as do snacks like pickles, crackers, peanuts, pretzels, chips, etc., so look for items that are labeled "low salt" or "no sodium added." Watch out for the food additive monosodium glutamate (MSG), which is high in sodium.

When signs of hepatic encephalopathy (mental confusion) appear, doctors may suggest a restriction of your animal protein intake, to be replaced by vegetable protein. (The types of protein in meat are more likely to promote hepatic encephalopathy.) They may also prescribe a medicine called lactulose, which helps to remove the buildup of proteins in the bowel that promotes encephalopathy. Before you restrict yourself from any kind of food, make sure you discuss this with your healthcare providers.

## Abstinence from Alcohol

Fred is a 45-year-old with chronic hepatitis C who has drunk five to ten beers daily over the last twenty years. After he was diagnosed with severe hepatitis, he was advised to abstain from alcohol to prevent further damage to his liver. He made the comment "What is life without alcohol?" and insisted that all his friends drank as much as he did, if not more.

Fred was advised that treatment for his hepatitis C could not be recommended as long as he continued to drink. After his condition had been monitored for two years by his doctor, and there had been no obvious improvement of his liver blood tests despite his efforts to cut back on his drinking, he was finally convinced that he needed help. He agreed to participate in an alcohol rehabilitation program. Fred has now been totally abstinent for a year and his liver enzymes have improved although, as expected, he still has hepatitis C. He is about to undergo a liver biopsy to assess the severity of his hepatitis C, now that he is no longer drinking.

Alcohol affects almost all organs of the body, especially the liver, the brain and the pancreas. Alcohol is almost completely eliminated from the body by the liver, and the amount of damage it does to the liver is related to the dose and duration of alcohol use. It is the alcohol content of the drink and not the type of beverage that is important in determining its effect. In fact, a bottle of beer, a glass of wine and a shot of liquor each contain about the same amount of alcohol, and all have the same effect on the liver.

The use of alcohol can result in an accumulation of fat in the liver cells, damage or death of liver cells and scarring of the liver. The degree of damage is proportional to the amount of alcohol consumed, but some people have liver damage with relatively low alcohol use while others have minimal effects despite prolonged and excessive alcohol consumption. Women are considerably more susceptible to the effects of alcohol than men.

Although the mechanism is not fully worked out, it is clear that there is an important interaction between alcohol use and the hepatitis C virus. It has been shown that people with hepatitis C are much more likely to develop severe liver damage if they drink alcohol (even in moderation) than if they abstain. Thus it is especially important that they not drink. In fact, for someone with chronic hepatitis C infection who drinks alcohol on a daily basis, the benefit of stopping

**What's a drink?**

All of the following are considered "one drink" and have approximately the same alcohol content.

- a 5 oz (142 mL) glass of wine (12 percent alcohol)
- a 12 oz (341 mL) bottle of beer (5 percent alcohol)
- a 1.5 oz (45 mL) shot of liquor (40 percent alcohol)
- a 3 oz (90 mL) glass of sherry or port (18 percent alcohol)

drinking may exceed the potential benefit of current drug treatment of the infection!

Many people believe that they are only "social drinkers," or that an excessive amount of alcohol consumed once in a while is not as harmful as drinking on a daily basis. However, if you have hepatitis C, binge drinking can be as bad as regular drinking. Alcohol not only prevents the growth of new liver cells, it actually increases the multiplication of the hepatitis C virus.

In addition, excessive drinking puts you at risk of getting any of several types of alcohol-induced liver disease. Recent studies have shown that even having less than three drinks per day increases your risk of getting more severe liver disease if you have hepatitis C. There is a clear association between the amount of alcohol drunk and the severity of the liver disease. How much drinking is too much? According to a consensus statement released by the National Institutes of Health in the U.S., people infected with hepatitis C *should not* have more than one drink per day, and no alcohol at all is recommended. This suggestion may seem difficult to go along with at first.

When you are under treatment with interferon for your hepatitis C, it is essential that you do not drink alcohol at all. A study has shown that alcohol intake *of any amount* decreases your chance of responding to treatment.

## Regular Exercise

A healthy lifestyle includes a regular exercise program. Walking at work or doing housework at home is not enough. Studies have shown that regular exercise helps to relieve symptoms of tiredness, stress and depression. If you are not already exercising, getting started with some friends is a good idea.

Your hepatitis C will not get worse with too little or too much exercise, but regular exercise will keep you in shape and build up your body's defenses. Listen to your body to determine how much exercise is enough; you do not want to exercise to the point that you feel you will collapse. Choose an exercise program that most suits your lifestyle and personality.

Suggested exercise activities include

- fast walking, biking, jogging, swimming, dancing
- low-impact aerobics or in-line or ice skating
- stationary machines such as treadmills, stair climbers, exercise bicycles
- tai chi, yoga

## Not Smoking

If in the years to come your liver starts to fail and a liver transplant is considered necessary, it will be vital that the rest of your body be in good shape. Smoking promotes the development of lung problems that would disqualify you from receiving a new liver. Smokers also seem to have more difficulty being weaned from the breathing machine that is necessary during the surgery. In addition, smoking promotes "hardening of the arteries" (arteriosclerosis), which may lead to a heart attack or a stroke—which would rule out a liver transplant. Hence, if you are a smoker, you need to overcome your habit.

# Positive Mental Outlook

Your regular exercise program will help you relax, but you might also consider taking a meditation class, or a course in relaxation techniques. Pace your daily activities to decrease your stress level. Cut down your intake of caffeine, from coffee, tea, cola and chocolate, to reduce any feeling of agitation. Take naps, if possible, to recharge your energy level. A healthy and relaxed mind will help you minimize symptoms like fatigue, poor appetite, sleep disturbance and depression.

# Your Work

One patient commented, "I can't work because I have cirrhosis." This idea is quite incorrect. A person with uncomplicated cirrhosis can be as productive as anyone else. If you do find full-time work is too tiring for you, look for part-time jobs. If you do not work outside your home, sign up for an interest course or volunteer your time to a social organization. You will find that you feel less worried about yourself when your time is occupied in a meaningful way.

In some workplaces, medical checkups are required before employment, and your hepatitis C status may be disclosed to your employer. However, confidentiality should be respected: your hepatitis C should not be made known to any other personnel. There are no work restrictions for people infected with hepatitis C. You may choose to talk to your co-workers about your condition, but it is wise to do so only if you feel they will be supportive.

Unfortunately this is not always the case, and you may be treated like a leper! Some co-workers refuse to shake hands with someone who has hepatitis C because they are afraid of catching the disease. A massage therapist may fear that he or she will become infected by touching a client with hepatitis C. We can only hope that, with better public education, such reactions will become rare. Moreover, there are cases where the employer and co-workers provide full support to the infected individual. This support is of the utmost importance if you go through a course of treatment, which may sometimes interfere with your work productivity.

## Networking

Social networking is a good way to reach out and get support from other people with the same problems. You can network through local or national hepatitis C support groups, public health seminars, newsletters and Internet chat groups. A strong social support network helps to improve your sense of well-being. However, some people prefer not to take this approach. They must then rely on family members or friends instead. A psychotherapist, social worker or private counselor can also be helpful when you need to ventilate your anger, anxiety, fear and other feelings associated with hepatitis C.

Joining a group for people with hepatitis C should help to keep you up-to-date on new information about the disease, and to give you insight into how to deal with different issues. The aim of such groups should be to make the disease easier to live with.

When you pick up new information through media sources, such as the newspaper and the Internet, it is important to distinguish good, reliable sources from dubious ones. Remember, information on the Internet is not always regulated or screened by experts, so be wary of non-credible claims for new therapies and remedies. When you are in doubt, check with your doctor, nurse or other healthcare professionals.

## Caution in Taking Prescribed and Over-the-Counter Medications

One of the functions of the liver is to detoxify drugs and harmful toxins by converting them into substances that can be excreted in the stools or urine. If you avoid any unnecessary drug intake, you are doing your liver a favor. The potentially harmful effects of some over-the-counter drugs should not be underestimated (see Chapter 5). There are also many prescribed medications that can harm the liver in certain individuals. Sometimes these harmful effects are predictable and other times they are not.

Acetaminophen in prescribed doses is quite safe in people with a liver problem of any degree. Only when it is taken in excess or in combination with alcohol does it become harmful to the liver. If you have cirrhosis, you should not take other painkillers such as ASA (called "aspirin" in the U.S.A.) or most arthritis pills, as these drugs may adversely affect your kidney function, and may promote variceal hemorrhage (internal bleeding in the esophagus and stomach).

Fortunately, most medications are in fact safe to use. However, you should not take any medication without checking with your doctor or pharmacist. It is also very important for you to know the names of all the medications you are taking, and why you are taking them. Write the names of all the drugs you are taking on a piece of paper, and carry this in your wallet at all times.

## Protection against Hepatitis A and B

When you have hepatitis C, it is recommended that you be vaccinated against hepatitis A and hepatitis B. One report from Italy has suggested that liver failure can be caused by acute hepatitis A in someone already infected with hepatitis C. Although the hepatitis A and B vaccine recommendation is not supported by all experts, it seems sensible to protect yourself this way.

A combined hepatitis A and hepatitis B vaccine is now available. It may be the vaccine of choice if you do not already have immunity to either of these two viruses. The combined vaccine is given in a course of three shots, with the second and third at one and six months from the day of the first shot. The vaccine will give you up to 98 percent protection against both viruses after the third dose. Side effects may include mild swelling, redness and soreness at the injection site. These are very common side effects and usually resolve in a few days.

Flu shots or pneumonia shots are generally recommended for people who have weak immune systems, such as the elderly and people with chronic diseases such as asthma. Some specialists also recommend these shots for individuals who have cirrhosis of the liver. You should discuss this with your family doctor, and decide whether you are a good candidate for these shots.

## Seeing a Liver Specialist

Ideally, everyone with hepatitis C should eventually see a liver specialist. But at present there are just not enough specialists to go around, and family doctors are becoming increasingly knowledgeable about hepatitis C and its management. If the liver enzyme count in your blood (ALT) is normal, your family doctor need only monitor it regularly. If and when the ALT level rises, you should be referred to a physician who has special expertise in the management of hepatitis. This can be a liver doctor (hepatologist), gastroenterologist or infectious-disease doctor. The specialist should be able to give you the most current treatments and up-to-date information on hepatitis C.

# E I G H T

# Complementary Therapies

any factors have caused an increase in the use of complementary (alternative) therapies over the last five years. One is clearly the public's dissatisfaction with therapies currently provided for certain health problems by the traditional medical profession. Hepatitis C is a good example.

The best understood of the alternative therapies are herbal remedies that have been used for over two millennia. Such treatments have, until recently, been used mostly in the Far East, where many different regimens have been tried but few have been tested by a modern "randomized control trial"— that is, comparing the effect of the herbal treatment with the effect of a placebo (dummy) pill, to make sure the herbal treatment actually helps. Only now are such trials being started. Some alternative medicines have been shown in the laboratory to have effects that can be beneficial in hepatitis C (as judged by a fall in the level of transaminases in the blood), but none has so far been shown to consistently cause a virus to stop multiplying and re-infecting liver cells.

## Dietary Supplements
You may be wondering, "Do I need to take vitamins or other supplements?" If you are eating a well-balanced diet with no

food restrictions, your body is getting enough nutrients from natural sources. Taking a multivitamin every day is certainly not harmful. However, you need to remember that some of the fat-soluble vitamins, such as A and D, are toxic when taken in excessive amounts. The small amount of vitamin A in a typical multivitamin is acceptable, but avoid taking a separate vitamin A supplement; a dose greater than 10,000 units per day can promote liver scarring.

> Marie is a 35-year-old executive who has known she has chronic hepatitis C for over ten years. She has received two courses of antiviral treatment but she is still infected. She was naturally very disappointed with the treatment results, and friends recommended she take herbal products, including milk thistle, garlic, St. John's wort, vitamin E and calcium. She is not sure exactly what these products will do to her health, yet she is convinced that her sense of well-being is improved. She feels that she needs to do something to help her liver, but sometimes she wonders if she is wasting her money.

Over the years, herbal supplements have become increasingly popular among people with chronic illnesses, in part because traditional medicine seems to have so little to offer, as has been the case for hepatitis C. The currently approved treatment with Rebetron has an overall success rate of only around 40 percent, and can cause a wide range of side effects. For those people who are not helped by this treatment, or who do not choose to or cannot take it, herbal remedies offer another option.

If you decide to buy herbal supplements, you need to realize that these products are not currently regulated in the same very strict manner as prescription drugs. Government agencies are in the process of improving the system of quality control. The ingredients in the product can vary from lot to lot, and it is not advisable to take a mixture of several herbs.

In general, people who take herbal remedies say that they feel an improvement in their sense of well-being. Unfortunately, to date there is no evidence that liver function is improved or that eradication of HCV RNA can be achieved using any complementary treatments. Whatever herbal substances you decide to take, it is always wise to inform your doctors, because some can be harmful.

## Herbs That Can Help

One herb that appears to have great potential benefit is glycyrrhizia (from the licorice root). Glycyrrhizia not only causes the level of transaminases in the blood to fall; it also affects the function of the lymphocytes, cells necessary for the eradication of viruses from the body. There is a report that glycyrrhizia may reduce the infectivity of both hepatitis B and hepatitis C. Unfortunately it has to be given intravenously. Because licorice root causes water retention, glycyrrhizia should not be taken by someone who already has cirrhosis.

Other herbs that are safe and may help are *Phyllanthus amarus* (said to help people with hepatitis B) and daphnoretin. Both have been shown in the laboratory to suppress the multiplication of hepatitis B (there have been no studies in hepatitis C). Tested in human cells in the laboratory, both appear to stimulate the body's natural antiviral machinery. But studies in human subjects are still needed.

Silymarin, the major extract from milk thistle, has become perhaps the herbal remedy most frequently used by those with liver disease. Silymarin has been shown in the laboratory to have a number of effects that could help a liver infected with hepatitis C. There is good evidence that it reduces the activity of the cells in the liver that produce scar tissue (fibrosis). Also, silymarin is a potent "scavenger" of damaging free radicals. (Another name for a "scavenger" is *antioxidant*.) Thus silymarin may protect the delicate linings of cells from damage caused by free radicals. A number of randomized control trials employing different herbs have been and are being conducted but the results to date are controversial. So far, there are indications that therapy with silymarin may improve survival in people with severe cirrhosis due to alcohol, and help those with an acute viral hepatitis or a liver severely damaged by a specific poisonous mushroom.

Picroliv—made from the root of *Picrorrhiza kurroa*, used mainly in India—has also been shown in rats to act as an antioxidant, and to reduce liver damage in rats fed specific agents that harm the liver, but well-documented studies in humans are lacking.

An agent known as TJ-9 in the West has been used in China (where it is called xiao-chai-hutang) and in Japan (sho-saiko-to); it also has antioxidant properties. TJ-9 is a mixture of herbs that include scutellaria, glycyrrhizia and bupleurum ginseng as well as pinella tuber, jujube fruit and the thew ginger rhizome. The effects of TJ-9 on the function of human cells in culture are claimed to be multiple—antioxidant and antibiotic effects, to name but two. One large study undertaken in Japan suggests that TJ-9 may improve the survival of people with cirrhosis, particularly those infected with hepatitis B.

Another mixture of ten herbs, known as compound 861, has long been part of traditional Chinese medicine. Non-randomized studies (studies without comparison to a placebo) suggest that compound 861 may reduce the formation of scar tissue in people with liver disease.

## Herbal Remedies to Avoid

A number of herbal remedies are toxic, often to the liver. Between 1991 and 1995, 785 reported cases were well documented in the U.S. Herbs to avoid are crotalaria, senecio, heliotropium, comfrey, *Atractylis gummifera*, *Callilepsis lau-*

## Herbal remedies that can be toxic

| | |
|---|---|
| Artemisia | Jin bu huang |
| *Atractylis gummifera* | LIV.52 |
| *Callilepsis laureola* | Ma huang |
| Chaparral leaf | Mistletoe |
| Chrysanthemum | Plantago seed |
| Comfrey | Red peony root |
| Crotalaria | Senecio |
| Gardenia | Skullcap |
| Germander | Valerian root |
| Greater celandine | |
| Hares' ear | |
| Heliotropium | |

*reola*, greater celandine, chaparral leaf, germander, artemisia, hares' ear, chrysanthemum, plantago seed, gardenia, red peony root, skullcap, valerian root, ma huang, jin bu huang, LIV.52 and mistletoe! Certain herbal teas have sometimes been found to be contaminated with toxic products, hence the advice not to buy anything that is sold as a mixture. A recent report suggests that even milk thistle may not always be innocuous; as with all medicines, unpredictable side effects may occur in some people.

## Homeopathy

Homeopathic medicine is based on the theory that taking minute amounts of agents that cause the same symptoms an individual complains of may give relief. There is no scientific proof of measurable benefit, but as the doses are very small, they are unlikely to be harmful.

## Non-Drug Therapies

It is not unusual for people with a chronic illness of any sort to have a number of non-specific symptoms for which "traditional" and even "alternate" remedies bring no relief. Many people report that these symptoms are sometimes relieved by exercises that promote relaxation and diminution of stress-related disorders. Some advocate one of the many types of massage therapy available. Others prefer to participate actively in activities such as yoga or tai chi. To each his own.

Everyone who delivers healthcare needs to keep in mind the benefits of a holistic approach. Too often, the details of "targeted" therapy are emphasized, while non-specific complaints receive less attention—mainly because so much less is known about them!

Currently it is unclear whether symptoms such as fatigue, poor concentration and the like—common complaints in people infected with the hepatitis C virus—are directly due to the virus infection or not. In any case, we need to do as much as possible to help these people take advantage of the many good things life has to offer—whether this is through the lifestyle changes described in Chapter 7, or through cautious use of complementary remedies, or through a broader range of stress-reducing therapies.

# NINE

*The Future
of Antiviral
Therapy*

## Other Interferons

There are three types of interferon: alpha, beta and gamma. (Some publications identify these by the Greek characters— α, β and γ, respectively.) Only the first two have been used in the treatment of hepatitis C. Because both IFN alpha and IFN beta are used to treat other diseases, there are several forms available on the market. Because ribavirin is not at present available on its own (but only with IFN alpha 2b, in Rebetron), combination therapy with interferons other than alpha 2b is not possible in Canada or the U.S.A. However, this is bound to change shortly.

There are situations when interferon alpha is safe alone but not if given in combination with ribavirin: for example, chronic renal (kidney) failure. Interferon alpha 2a (Roferon) has not been compared head-to-head with IFN alpha 2b (Intron A) so it is not known if they are equally effective. But interferon alpha-con-1 (Infergen) has been compared with Intron A and overall they are comparable, although Infergen is more effective than Intron A when the level of the hepatitis C virus in the blood is very high.

## Induction Therapy

One of the reasons why the cure rate of hepatitis C is so low when IFN therapy is given alone is that the intermittent dosing allows the virus to rebound in the blood between doses. Therefore it has been suggested that treatment should be given daily and in high doses (induction therapy) for the first few weeks of therapy. To the surprise of everyone, daily dosing is not associated with more side effects, although higher doses are. But although there is a higher chance of clearing HCV RNA from the blood during induction treatment, the relapse rate is high, so overall there appears to be little or no advantage to daily dosing of IFN.

## Pegylated Interferons

If interferon is combined with an inert substance (polyethylene glycol, a substance present in many foodstuffs), the absorption of the IFN from the injection site is delayed. As well, the excretion of the IFN is markedly delayed, so that high levels of IFN remain in the blood for over a week (standard IFN lasts in the blood for no more than sixteen hours). Several forms of combined or "pegylated" interferons have been developed and evaluated in people infected with hepatitis C; one was licensed in the U.S.A. in 2001, and others will soon be licensed. The results from trials are very promising. Side effects are no more than with standard IFN given intermittently, but are 50 percent less than with Rebetron. The rate of loss of HCV RNA seems comparable to that with Rebetron, but the two drugs have not been compared head-to-head.

Trials are currently ongoing combining pegylated interferons with ribavirin, in the hope that an even greater rate of viral eradication will be achieved. However, it is expected that once pegylated IFN is combined with ribavirin, the side effects will be greater than when pegylated interferon is used alone.

## Combining Alpha Interferons with Other Agents

A number of studies have tested whether the effectiveness of alpha IFNs can be increased by combining them with other agents, such as amantadine, ursodeoxycholic acid, non-steroidal anti-inflammatory agents (NSAIDs) and thymosin alpha. Trials where IFN alpha alone has been compared with IFN alpha and one or more of these other drugs show no increase in the rate of viral eradication. But when Rebetron was combined with amantadine, some (but not all) studies indicated additional benefit, although more side effects were noted.

## Future Treatments for Hepatitis C

The best treatment available at the present time, namely Rebetron, leads to permanent loss of the hepatitis C virus in less than half of those who receive a full course of therapy. As many as 21 percent have to stop Rebetron therapy because the side effects become intolerable. Clearly there is much room for improvement in the medical therapy of hepatitis C.

New approaches are being developed. Initially there was much enthusiasm about the possibility of developing drugs similar to those that have been so successful in treating AIDS: protease inhibitors. But these kinds of drugs are proving to be much more difficult to develop for hepatitis C because of the very different structure of the hepatitis C virus. So other approaches are being explored.

There are potentially several other ways in which the multiplication of this virus could be brought to a halt. Agents called *ribozymes* and others called *antisense oligonucleotides* are already in development, but before trials are conducted in humans we need to be certain that these drugs will attack only the genetic material (RNA) of the hepatitis C virus, and not that of the person.

Ribavirin improves the effectiveness of alpha interferons in several ways but, given on its own, it does not prevent hepatitis C virus from multiplying. But ribavirin does inhibit an important protein needed in the manufacture of HCV RNA. This protein is called *inosine monophosphate dehydrogenase* (IMPDH). Recently a more effective IMPDH inhibitor has been developed. It appears that when this is given alone to humans it is safe—but, like ribavirin, when it is given alone it does not cause levels of virus to fall in the blood. It too will likely need to be combined with an IFN to effectively eradicate hepatitis C.

## Modulation of the Immune Response

It is probable that ribavirin works mostly by stimulating the immune system to fight the hepatitis C virus more aggressively. But if trying to stimulate the immune system fails, an alternative approach has been tried: reduce the immune response to the virus, and thus reduce the damage it causes to liver cells. Early studies have shown that the cytokine IL-10 may just do this. It does not do anything to clear the virus, but it reduces the liver damage and fibrosis (scar tissue) caused by the hepatitis C infection.

## A Vaccine for Hepatitis C?

There are vaccines that work very well at protecting us from both hepatitis A and hepatitis B. In both these diseases, protective antibodies develop during the infection and increase in amount once the virus is eradicated. Whether these antibodies develop naturally or are a result of vaccination, they protect us from ever being infected again.

But we know from human studies that, even though the hepatitis C virus can be spontaneously lost or eradicated by antiviral therapy, re-infection is possible. It seems that there are no natural, long-lasting protective antibodies against hepatitis C. Thus we will have to take very different approaches to develop a vaccine for hepatitis C. Also, it will have to protect us from not just one but all the different geno-types. This is currently a very active area of research, and if it is successful it will have a marked benefit for people the world over. Let us hope we don't have to wait too long!

Also in development are vaccines that can be used to treat people already infected with hepatitis C. These would work by stimulating the person's own immune system to eradicate the virus. Such vaccines are already being used to treat people infected with hepatitis B.

# T E N

## How Can Others Help?

If you have a friend or family member with hepatitis C, by reading this book you have taken an important step toward helping. To be effective in assisting someone who has hepatitis C, which may become a lifelong disease, you may want to know about the different stages of grieving an individual goes through in coping with a loss, as discussed in Chapter 3: shock and denial, understanding the disease, attempting to deal with it and final resolution. Having chronic hepatitis C is a health loss to your friend. By understanding these stages of coping, you can assist your friend in living with the infection.

## Dealing with Shock and Denial

At this stage your presence as a friend is precious. You may want to let the person know that you are there to help. It is not a good idea to confront your friend with the diagnosis at this time, and force him or her to accept the truth. Do not make any judgment about how your friend should feel or deal with the disease right now; it is too early to do that. He or she needs to be able to express anger. You may want to encourage your friend to talk about the problem, to go for a walk or have a good workout. At this point it is important to apply angry energy in a positive and useful direction.

People with hepatitis C sometimes become depressed knowing that they have a chronic disease, that they are carrying a virus, and they may become afraid to keep in touch with others. So it is essential for you to keep up regular contact.

In addition, it helps if you know about the causes, transmission and available treatments. For example, some people say that hepatitis C is like AIDS, which is still a very dangerous virus. Such misinformation could even cause someone infected with hepatitis C to have thoughts of ending his or her life, to avoid transmitting the disease to others or becoming a burden.

Pay extra attention if you think your friend is having suicidal thoughts. If you suspect that suicide is a possibility, you should strongly urge professional help. If, after assessing your friend, the family doctor concludes that this person is indeed at risk of suicide, the doctor is legally bound to get the help of a psychiatrist or psychologist immediately.

By spending time listening to your friend and sharing worries, you can help to correct the myths about hepatitis C. As a friend, you should try to get information that will help both of you deal with this diagnosis. However, your friend may need you to make the first move: that is, to take the initiative in finding people with the same diagnosis, and doctors who can give further information, advice and support.

Mary was devastated to find out that she had hepatitis C, and that she had probably been infected for a long time—ever since experimenting with injected street drugs in her youth, some ten years earlier. She was told that she would have this disease for the rest of her life. Mary assumed that the terms "hepatitis" and "lifelong disease" meant that she was going to die soon. She became very depressed and withdrawn. She did not want to communicate with others, even her roommate, Diana. This was very upsetting for Diana because they had been good friends for years. Mary started to lose weight, which scared her even more.

Diana ignored Mary until one day she caught her crying in bed. Mary would not say anything at first, but she cried more and more. Eventually she opened up and talked about her diagnosis. Diana did not know what to say at the time, but she sat and listened to Mary talk about her feelings and was alarmed to hear that Mary thought she was going to die. It did not matter how much Diana encouraged her to seek help, Mary would not go.

Diana knew nothing about hepatitis C, so she started looking for references, and she contacted the Liver Foundation to get more information. After doing some research on hepatitis C, Diana managed to convince Mary that she was not about to die, and that there was treatment that could suppress the activity of the virus and reduce any damage to her liver. Eventually Mary decided to seek support, after Diana convinced her that both professional help and support groups were available to assist her.

## Understanding the Disease

It is difficult to pass through the stage of shock and denial, but with your support your friend will accept the fact of hepatitis C infection and become interested in learning more about it. You may recognize that he or she has entered this stage if the talk turns to facing the reality of the diagnosis. This is when your friend has the ability to experience and express painful feelings and worries. Whatever the situation, you just need to be there to listen. At this stage he or she may be ready to learn more about the disease, so it may be helpful if you are available to discuss issues your friend is not sure about, such as decisions regarding the treatment options. However, it is very important that you not give any opinion about a treatment unless you are well informed and understand the pros and cons. To help yourself learn more about treatment, you could accompany your friend to as many clinic visits with the doctor or nurse as possible—that is, if your presence is welcome.

Tears may be shed at this stage. This is a good sign, although you may find it somewhat embarrassing! Tell your friend that this is a normal and expected response, but gently remind the person of reality, and encourage him or her to find out more about what can be done, *right now*, to help stop or slow down the damage that hepatitis C can cause. Once both of you know the facts, your friend should feel more comfortable about dealing with the infection.

As a healthy 34-year-old, John decided to donate blood. He was very surprised to be informed by letter that he had tested positive for hepatitis C. In fact, he was shocked!

John had a steady girlfriend, Simone, whom he planned to marry in a year or so. Upon hearing the news, he decided to break up with Simone, because he did not want to infect her and any children they might have. He became very depressed and isolated. Simone didn't understand why John wanted to break up but, instead of getting upset, she recognized that he was very depressed. She tried to talk to him to see if there were any specific problems, but John did not admit that anything was wrong. However, Simone had called him at work and knew that John had taken several sick days. After she asked him many times, he finally talked about his hepatitis C.

Willing to support John, Simone volunteered to go with him to his doctors' appointments. After learning more about hepatitis C at the doctor's office, and reading books on the disease, she became best friends with John once more. She was very involved with his treatment, and made sure that he kept it up. She planned activities and prepared a proper lunch and dinner with lots of fluid and fruit. With her support, and his newly learned knowledge about the transmission of hepatitis C and its progression, John was able to accept his diagnosis. He managed to deal with it effectively, and started to live a normal life as before. Before long, John and Simone were planning their wedding.

## Attempting to Deal with the Disease

At this stage, your friend should seek further information on the disease by talking with healthcare professionals or other people with hepatitis C—perhaps with you in tow. Once all the information is gathered and analyzed, you should be able to develop a positive approach to therapy. While your friend is on a treatment, it is important that he or she acknowledge all the side effects, so that you can help in dealing with them.

If there are flu-like symptoms, you can remind your friend of the importance of eating a well-balanced diet, drinking plenty of water, exercising regularly and trying hard to be as productive as possible. If your friend is tired and not interested in cooking, it will be very helpful if you can prepare food and encourage regular meal and fluid intake; he or she should drink at least two to three quarts (liters) of fluid per day.

Psychological support plays a major role while someone is on interferon treatment. Irritability and depression are two common side effects experienced, to varying degrees, by many people. Often the person will deny these symptoms. Instead of getting upset with your friend's treatment-induced anger, it may be advisable to contact the doctor or nurse as soon as possible. If unusual behaviors are noticed and reported, the problem can be dealt with right away, before any unacceptable behavior takes place—for example, fighting with others or having ideas of self-destruction. The treating doctor and nurse are available to monitor your friend, but they will not always be able to identify unusual behaviors at the time of a regular clinic visit.

Some people use alcohol to cope with their symptoms, especially if they have been heavy drinkers in the past. The alcohol is taken to forget the bad mood and the other side effects of interferon. Not only is alcohol harmful to general health, but it does not reduce the severity of the side effects, and it reduces the effectiveness of the treatment and damages the liver further. *All alcohol consumption should be discouraged.*

## Final Resolution

If your friend learns that he or she is a non-responder or a relapser, this news can be very upsetting. He or she may feel that time, energy and money have been wasted, and may need a good listener to pay attention to these feelings. Be supportive by sending a message that there will be other treatments available in the future. It also helps to continue pointing out your friend's strengths, particularly after he or she has put so much effort into the treatment regimen.

Encourage your friend to continue to follow up with the doctor, so that the liver disease is monitored and the doctor knows when other measures have to be taken. An additional benefit is that your friend will be kept informed of any new treatments as they become available.

What do you do if your friend has successfully responded to treatment? Share the happiness!

# Drugs and the Treatment of Hepatitis C

| Antiviral medications | |
|---|---|
| Generic | Brand |
| interferon alpha 2a | Roferon |
| interferon alpha 2b | Intron A |
| interferon alpha-con-1 | Infergen |
| interferon alpha 2b + ribavirin | Rebetron |
| **Drugs for relief of symptoms** | |
| Generic | Some common brand names |
| acetaminophen | Atasol†, Tempra, Tylenol |
| dimenhydrinate | Dramamine*, Gravol† |
| lactulose | Acilac, Lactulax |
| **Benzodiazepines—to be avoided** | |
| Generic | Some common brand names |
| diazepam | Valium |
| lorazepam | Ativan |
| oxazepam | Serax |

\* U.S. only
† Canada only

# Glossary

**ALT:** alanine aminotransferase, an enzyme present in liver cells which gets into the bloodstream when the cell is damaged; *see* **Transaminases.**

**ASA:** acetylsalicylic acid, also called aspirin in the U.S.A. (In Canada, "Aspirin" is a brand name.)

**Ascites:** accumulation of fluid in abdomen.

**AST:** aspartate aminotransferase, similar to ALT, above.

**Bile:** a fluid produced by the liver and used in the process of digestion. Bile is stored in the gallbladder until it is needed.

**Bile duct:** duct that drains bile from the liver and delivers it to the duodenum; part of the biliary system. *See also* **Bile.**

**Biliary system:** a series of ducts which drain bile made in the liver into the gastrointestinal tract.

**Cirrhosis:** scar tissue that surrounds and isolates liver cells, seriously affecting liver function and the flow of blood through the liver.

**Cryoglobulinemia:** a complication of hepatitis C which can cause a variety of symptoms (arthritis, skin rashes, nerve and kidney problems).

**Diuretic:** a medication that causes the kidneys to excrete more salt and water into the urine.

**Encephalopathy:** mental confusion.

**Extrahepatic:** outside the liver.

**Fibrosis:** scar tissue.

**Gastroscopy:** examination of the gastrointestinal tract with the aid of an illuminated tube.

**Genotype:** a group of closely related virus sequences. There are at least six different major genotypes of the hepatitis C virus, and they vary somewhat in their biological properties, including susceptibility to antiviral therapy.

**HCV:** hepatitis C virus. *See also* **RNA**.

**Hemolysis:** premature destruction of red blood cells, causing the blood count to fall.

**Hepatic artery:** artery bringing oxygen-bearing blood from the heart to the liver.

**Hepatitis:** inflammation of the liver. The main forms of hepatitis are caused by viruses designated by letters (A, B, C etc.), but there are many other causes of liver inflammation, such as alcohol and toxic reactions to medications.

**Hepatocyte:** liver cell.

**Hepatologist:** liver specialist.

**IFN:** *see* **Interferon**.

**Interferon (IFN):** a kind of protein used to treat viral infections. There are different kinds of interferon.

**Jaundice:** yellowing of the whites of the eyes.

**Lobe:** one of the two halves of the liver (right lobe and left lobe). The lobes are divided into eight smaller sections composed of millions of lobules, which are made up of many kinds of cells with different functions.

**Lobule:** *see* **Lobe**.

**Lymphocyte:** a white blood cell that is particularly important in fighting off infection with a virus.

**Non-responder:** *see* **Responder**.

**Portal tracts:** areas between the lobules of the liver. The portal vein, hepatic artery and bile duct all pass through the portal tracts.

**Portal vein:** vein bringing blood from the intestines to the liver, where nutrients will pass to the liver and toxins will be filtered out.

**Prothrombin time:** the time it takes blood to clot—measured in seconds.

**Responder:** someone whose hepatitis is cured by antiviral medication; in some people (non-responders) the medication is not effective.

**RNA:** the genetic material ribonucleic acid. If the RNA for hepatitis C virus (HCV RNA) shows up in someone's blood, it means the person is infected with this virus.

**Septicemia:** bacterial infection of the blood (circulatory) system.

**Transaminases:** enzymes in liver cells that spill over into the blood when there is damage to the liver cells. The level of transaminases in the blood is a rough guide to the degree of liver-cell damage occurring on the day of the blood test.

**Variceal hemorrhage:** rupturing of dilated veins in the esophagus and stomach of someone with cirrhosis of the liver. This results in vomiting of blood with or without the passage of black bowel movements.

**Viral load:** the concentration of virus in someone's blood.

**Virus:** an infectious organism that requires the "machinery" of the cells of the body to multiply.

# *Further Resources*

## Organizations

### *U.S.A.*

American Liver Foundation
75 Maiden Lane, Suite 603
New York, NY  10038-4810
Toll-free: 1-800-223-0179
(212)668-1000
www.liverfoundation.org

Centers for Disease Control
  and Prevention (CDC)
Hepatitis Branch
1600 Clifton Road
Atlanta, GA  30333
Toll-free (U.S. only):
  1-888-443-7232
www.cdc.gov/hepatitis

Hepatitis Foundation
  International
30 Sunrise Terrace
Cedar Grove, NJ  07009
Toll-free: 1-800-891-0707
www.hepfi.org

## Canada

Canadian Hemophilia
  Society
625 President Kennedy Ave.
Suite 1210
Montreal, PQ  H3A 1K2
Toll-free: 1-800-668-2686
(514)848-0503
Fax: (514)848-9661
E-mail: chs@hemophilia.ca
www.hemophilia.ca

Hepatitis C Society of
  Canada
3050 Confederation
  Parkway, Suite 301B
Mississauga, ON  L5B 3Z6
Toll-free (outside Toronto):
  1-800-652-4372
(905)270-1110
www.hepatitiscsociety.com

Canadian Liver Foundation
2235 Sheppard Avenue E.
Suite 1500
Toronto, ON  M2J 5B5
Toll-free: 1-800-563-5483
(416)491-3353
E-mail: clf@liver.ca
www.liver.ca

### Other Internet Sites

HCV Global Foundation, *www.hcvglobal.org*

Hepatitis Information Network (sponsored by
  Schering Canada), *www.hepnet.com*

Hepatitis Magazine, *www.hepatitismag.com*
  (tel: 1-800-310-7047)

Hep-C Alert, *www.hep-c-alert.org*
  (tel: 877-HELP-4-HEP [877-435-7443])

HIV and Hepatitis Information,
  *www.HIVandHepatitis.com*

Parents of Kids with Infectious Diseases (PKIDS),
  *www.pkids.org* (tel: 877-557-5437)

## Books

Cohen, Misha, and Robert Gish, with Kalia Doner. *The Hepatitis C Help Book*. New York, NY: St. Martin's, 2000.

Dolan, Matthew. *The Hepatitis C Handbook*. London, England: Catalyst, 1997.

Everson, Gregory, with Hedy Weinberg. *Living with Hepatitis C: A Survivor's Guide*. New York, NY: Hatherleigh, 1997.

Kennedy, Sidney, Sagar Parikh and Colin Shapiro. *Defeating Depression*. Thornhill, ON: Joli Joco, 1998.

Petro Roybal, Beth Ann. *Hepatitis C: A Personal Guide to Good Health*. Berkeley, CA: Ulysses, 1997.

Shapiro, Colin, James MacFarlane and Mohamed Hussain. *Conquering Insomnia*. Hamilton, ON: Empowering, 1994.

Weil, Andrew. *Spontaneous Healing: Discover and Enhance Your Body's Natural Ability to Maintain and Heal Itself*. New York: Random House, 1995.

# Index

Page numbers in italic indicate a figure. For drug brands please see the table of drug names on page 119.